Steven Godin, PhD, MPH, CHES
Editor

Technology Applications in Prevention

Technology Applications in Prevention has been co-published simultaneously as *Journal of Prevention & Intervention in the Community*, Volume 29, Numbers 1/2 2005.

Pre-publication
REVIEWS,
COMMENTARIES,
EVALUATIONS . . .

"MUCH-NEEDED. . . . Can move us closer toward building models that harness technology for improved efficacy in prevention efforts. The spectrum of applications in this book is logically arrayed along a continuum of care directed toward initiatives for community health–from local to international levels."

Joseph S. Coyne, DrPH
Professor
Department of Health Policy &
Administration
Director
Center for International Health
Services Research & Policy
Washington State University

Technology Applications in Prevention

Technology Applications in Prevention has been co-published simultaneously as *Journal of Prevention & Intervention in the Community*, Volume 29, Numbers 1/2 2005.

The *Journal of Prevention & Intervention in the Community*™ Monographic "Separates" (formerly the *Prevention in Human Services* series)*

For information on previous issues of *Prevention in Human Services*, edited by Robert E. Hess, please contact: The Haworth Press, Inc., 10 Alice Street, Binghamton, NY 13904-1580 USA.

Below is a list of "separates," which in serials librarianship means a special issue simultaneously published as a special journal issue or double-issue *and* as a "separate" hardbound monograph. (This is a format which we also call a "DocuSerial.")

"Separates" are published because specialized libraries or professionals may wish to purchase a specific thematic issue by itself in a format which can be separately cataloged and shelved, as opposed to purchasing the journal on an on-going basis. Faculty members may also more easily consider a "separate" for classroom adoption.

"Separates" are carefully classified separately with the major book jobbers so that the journal tie-in can be noted on new book order slips to avoid duplicate purchasing.

You may wish to visit Haworth's website at . . .

http://www.HaworthPress.com

. . . to search our online catalog for complete tables of contents of these separates and related publications.

You may also call 1-800-HAWORTH (outside US/Canada: 607-722-5857), or Fax 1-800-895-0582 (outside US/Canada: 607-771-0012), or e-mail at:

docdelivery@haworthpress.com

Technology Applications in Prevention, edited by Steven Godin, PhD, MPH, CHES (Vol. 29, No. 1/2, 2005). *Examines new prevention options made possible by today's cutting-edge technology.*

Six Community Psychologists Tell Their Stories: History, Contexts, and Narrative, edited by James G. Kelly, PhD, and Anna V. Song, MA (Vol. 28, No. 1/2, 2004). *"Should be required reading for any student aspiring to become a community psychologist as well as for practicing community psychologists interested in being provided unparalleled insights into the personal stories of many of the leading figures within our field. This book provides readers with an inside look at the reasons why a second generation of community psychologists entered this field, and also provides a rare glimpse of the excitement and passion that occured at some of the most important and dynamic community training settings over the past 40 years." (Leonard A. Jason, PhD, Professor of Psychology and Director, Center for Community Research, DePaul University)*

Understanding Ecological Programming: Merging Theory, Research, and Practice, edited by Susan Scherffius Jakes, PhD, and Craig C. Brookins, PhD (Vol. 27, No. 2, 2004). *Examines the background, concept, components, and benefits of using ecological programming in intervention/ prevention program designs.*

Leadership and Organization for Community Prevention and Intervention in Venezuela, edited by Maritza Montero, PhD (Vol. 27, No. 1, 2004). *Shows how (and why) participatory communities come into being, what they can accomplish, and how to help their leaders develop the skills they need to be most effective.*

Empowerment and Participatory Evaluation of Community Interventions: Multiple Benefits, edited by Yolanda Suarez-Balcazar, PhD, and Gary W. Harper, PhD, MPH (Vol. 26, No. 2, 2003). *"Useful . . . . Draws together diverse chapters that uncover the how and why of empowerment and participatory evaluation while offering exemplary case studies showing the challenges and successes of this community value-based evaluation model." (Anne E. Brodsky, PhD, Associate Professor of Psychology, University of Maryland Baltimore County)*

Traumatic Stress and Its Aftermath: Cultural, Community, and Professional Contexts, edited by Sandra S. Lee, PhD (Vol. 26, No. 1, 2003). *Explores risk and protective factors for traumatic stress, emphasizing the impact of cumulative/multiple trauma in a variety of populations, including therapists themselves.*

Culture, Peers, and Delinquency, edited by Clifford O'Donnell, PhD (Vol. 25, No. 2, 2003). *"Timely . . . of value to both students and professionals. . . . Demonstrates how peers can serve as a pathway to delinquency from a multiethnic perspective. The discussion of ethnic, racial, and gender differences challenges the field to reconsider assessment, treatment, and preventative approaches." (Donald Meichenbaum, PhD, Distinguished Professor Emeritus, University of Waterloo, Ontario, Canada; Research Director, The Melissa Institute for Violence Prevention and the Treatment of Victims of Violence, Miami, Florida)*

Prevention and Intervention Practice in Post-Apartheid South Africa, edited by Vijé Franchi, PhD, and Norman Duncan, PhD, consulting editor (Vol. 25, No.1, 2003). *"Highlights the way in which preventive and curative interventions serve–or do not serve–the ideals of equality, empowerment, and participation. . . . Revolutionizes our way of thinking about and teaching socio-pedagogical action in the context of exclusion." (Dr. Altay A. Manço, Scientific Director, Institute of Research, Training, and Action on Migrations, Belgium)*

Community Interventions to Create Change in Children, edited by Lorna H. London, PhD (Vol. 24, No. 2, 2002). *"Illustrates creative approaches to prevention and intervention with at-risk youth. . . . Describes multiple methods to consider in the design, implementation, and evaluation of programs." (Susan D. McMahon, PhD, Assistant Professor, Department of Psychology, DePaul University)*

Preventing Youth Access to Tobacco, edited by Leonard A. Jason, PhD, and Steven B. Pokorny, PhD (Vol. 24, No. 1, 2002). *"Explores cutting-edge issues in youth access research methodology. . . . Provides a thorough review of the tobacco control literature and detailed analysis of the methodological issues presented by community interventions to increase the effectiveness of tobacco control. . . . Challenges widespread assumptions about the dynamics of youth access programs and the requirements for long-term success." (John A. Gardiner, PhD, LLB, Consultant to the 2000 Surgeon General's Report* Reducing Youth Access to Tobacco *and to the National Cancer Institute's evaluation of the ASSIST program)*

The Transition from Welfare to Work: Processes, Challenges, and Outcomes, edited by Sharon Telleen, PhD, and Judith V. Sayad (Vol. 23, No. 1/2, 2002). *A comprehensive examination of the welfare-to-work initiatives surrounding the major reform of United States welfare legislation in 1996.*

Prevention Issues for Women's Health in the New Millennium, edited by Wendee M. Wechsberg, PhD (Vol. 22, No. 2, 2001). *"Helpful to service providers as well as researchers . . . A useful ancillary textbook for courses addressing women's health issues. Covers a wide range of health issues affecting women." (Sherry Deren, PhD, Director, Center for Drug Use and HIV Research, National Drug Research Institute, New York City)*

Workplace Safety: Individual Differences in Behavior, edited by Alice F. Stuhlmacher, PhD, and Douglas F. Cellar, PhD (Vol. 22, No. 1, 2001). Workplace Safety: Individual Differences in Behavior *examines safety behavior and outlines practical interventions to help increase safety awareness. Individual differences are relevant to a variety of settings, including the workplace, public spaces, and motor vehicles. This book takes a look at ways of defining and measuring safety as well as a variety of individual differences like gender, job knowledge, conscientiousness, self-efficacy, risk avoidance, and stress tolerance that are important in creating safety interventions and improving the selection and training of employees.* Workplace Safety *takes an incisive look at these issues with a unique focus on the way individual differences in people impact safety behavior in the real world.*

People with Disabilities: Empowerment and Community Action, edited by Christopher B. Keys, PhD, and Peter W. Dowrick, PhD (Vol. 21, No. 2, 2001). *"Timely and useful . . . provides valuable lessons and guidance for everyone involved in the disability movement. This book is a must-read for researchers and practitioners interested in disability rights issues!" (Karen M. Ward, EdD, Director, Center for Human Development; Associate Professor, University of Alaska, Anchorage)*

Family Systems/Family Therapy: Applications for Clinical Practice, edited by Joan D. Atwood, PhD (Vol. 21, No. 1, 2001). *Examines family therapy issues in the context of the larger systems of health, law, and education and suggests ways family therapists can effectively use an intersystems approach.*

HIV/AIDS Prevention: Current Issues in Community Practice, edited by Doreen D. Salina, PhD (Vol. 19, No. 1, 2000). *Helps researchers and psychologists explore specific methods of improving HIV/AIDS prevention research.*

Educating Students to Make-a-Difference: Community-Based Service Learning, edited by Joseph R. Ferrari, PhD, and Judith G. Chapman, PhD (Vol. 18, No. 1/2, 1999). *"There is something here for everyone interested in the social psychology of service-learning." (Frank Bernt, PhD, Associate Professor, St. Joseph's University)*

Program Implementation in Preventive Trials, edited by Joseph A. Durlak and Joseph R. Ferrari, PhD (Vol. 17, No. 2, 1998). *"Fills an important gap in preventive research. . . . Highlights an array of important questions related to implementation and demonstrates just how good community-based intervention programs can be when issues related to implementation are taken seriously." (Judy Primavera, PhD, Associate Professor of Psychology, Fairfield University, Fairfield, Connecticut)*

Preventing Drunk Driving, edited by Elsie R. Shore, PhD, and Joseph R. Ferrari, PhD (Vol. 17, No. 1, 1998). *"A must read for anyone interested in reducing the needless injuries and death caused by the drunk driver." (Terrance D. Schiavone, President, National Commission Against Drunk Driving, Washington, DC)*

Manhood Development in Urban African-American Communities, edited by Roderick J. Watts, PhD, and Robert J. Jagers (Vol. 16, No. 1/2, 1998). *"Watts and Jagers provide the much-needed foundational and baseline information and research that begins to philosophically and empirically validate the importance of understanding culture, oppression, and gender when working with males in urban African-American communities." (Paul Hill, Jr., MSW, LISW, ACSW, East End Neighborhood House, Cleveland, Ohio)*

Diversity Within the Homeless Population: Implications for Intervention, edited by Elizabeth M. Smith, PhD, and Joseph R. Ferrari, PhD (Vol. 15, No. 2, 1997). *"Examines why homelessness is increasing, as well as treatment options, case management techniques, and community intervention programs that can be used to prevent homelessness." (American Public Welfare Association)*

Education in Community Psychology: Models for Graduate and Undergraduate Programs, edited by Clifford R. O'Donnell, PhD, and Joseph R. Ferrari, PhD (Vol. 15, No. 1, 1997). *"An invaluable resource for students seeking graduate training in community psychology . . . [and will] also serve faculty who want to improve undergraduate teaching and graduate programs." (Marybeth Shinn, PhD, Professor of Psychology and Coordinator, Community Doctoral Program, New York University, New York, New York)*

Adolescent Health Care: Program Designs and Services, edited by John S. Wodarski, PhD, Marvin D. Feit, PhD, and Joseph R. Ferrari, PhD (Vol. 14, No. 1/2, 1997). *Devoted to helping practitioners address the problems of our adolescents through the use of preventive interventions based on sound empirical data.*

Preventing Illness Among People with Coronary Heart Disease, edited by John D. Piette, PhD, Robert M. Kaplan, PhD, and Joseph R. Ferrari, PhD (Vol. 13, No. 1/2, 1996). *"A useful contribution to the interaction of physical health, mental health, and the behavioral interventions for patients with CHD." (Public Health: The Journal of the Society of Public Health)*

Sexual Assault and Abuse: Sociocultural Context of Prevention, edited by Carolyn F. Swift, PhD* (Vol. 12, No. 2, 1995). *"Delivers a cornucopia for all who are concerned with the primary prevention of these damaging and degrading acts." (George J. McCall, PhD, Professor of Sociology and Public Administration, University of Missouri)*

International Approaches to Prevention in Mental Health and Human Services, edited by Robert E. Hess, PhD, and Wolfgang Stark* (Vol. 12, No. 1, 1995). *Increases knowledge of prevention strategies from around the world.*

Self-Help and Mutual Aid Groups: International and Multicultural Perspectives, edited by Francine Lavoie, PhD, Thomasina Borkman, PhD, and Benjamin Gidron* (Vol. 11, No. 1/2, 1995). *"A helpful orientation and overview, as well as useful data and methodological suggestions." (International Journal of Group Psychotherapy)*

Prevention and School Transitions, edited by Leonard A. Jason, PhD, Karen E. Danner, and Karen S. Kurasaki, MA* (Vol. 10, No. 2, 1994). *"A collection of studies by leading ecological and systems-oriented theorists in the area of school transitions, describing the stressors, personal re-*

sources available, and coping strategies among different groups of children and adolescents undergoing school transitions." (Reference & Research Book News)

Religion and Prevention in Mental Health: Research, Vision, and Action, edited by Kenneth I. Pargament, PhD, Kenneth I. Maton, PhD, and Robert E. Hess, PhD* (Vol. 9, No. 2 & Vol. 10, No. 1, 1992). *"The authors provide an admirable framework for considering the important, yet often overlooked, differences in theological perspectives." (Family Relations)*

Families as Nurturing Systems: Support Across the Life Span, edited by Donald G. Unger, PhD, and Douglas R. Powell, PhD* (Vol. 9, No. 1, 1991). *"A useful book for anyone thinking about alternative ways of delivering a mental health service." (British Journal of Psychiatry)*

Ethical Implications of Primary Prevention, edited by Gloria B. Levin, PhD, and Edison J. Trickett, PhD* (Vol. 8, No. 2, 1991). *"A thoughtful and thought-provoking summary of ethical issues related to intervention programs and community research." (Betty Tableman, MPA, Director, Division. of Prevention Services and Demonstration Projects, Michigan Department of Mental Health, Lansing) Here is the first systematic and focused treatment of the ethical implications of primary prevention practice and research.*

Career Stress in Changing Times, edited by James Campbell Quick, PhD, MBA, Robert E. Hess, PhD, Jared Hermalin, PhD, and Jonathan D. Quick, MD* (Vol. 8, No. 1, 1990). *"A well-organized book. . . . It deals with planning a career and career changes and the stresses involved." (American Association of Psychiatric Administrators)*

Prevention in Community Mental Health Centers, edited by Robert E. Hess, PhD, and John Morgan, PhD* (Vol. 7, No. 2, 1990). *"A fascinating bird's-eye view of six significant programs of preventive care which have survived the rise and fall of preventive psychiatry in the U.S." (British Journal of Psychiatry)*

Protecting the Children: Strategies for Optimizing Emotional and Behavioral Development, edited by Raymond P. Lorion, PhD* (Vol. 7, No. 1, 1990). *"This is a masterfully conceptualized and edited volume presenting theory-driven, empirically based, developmentally oriented prevention." (Michael C. Roberts, PhD, Professor of Psychology, The University of Alabama)*

The National Mental Health Association: Eighty Years of Involvement in the Field of Prevention, edited by Robert E. Hess, PhD, and Jean DeLeon, PhD* (Vol. 6, No. 2, 1989). *"As a family life educator interested in both the history of the field, current efforts, and especially the evaluation of programs, I find this book quite interesting. I enjoyed reviewing it and believe that I will return to it many times. It is also a book I will recommend to students." (Family Relations)*

A Guide to Conducting Prevention Research in the Community: First Steps, by James G. Kelly, PhD, Nancy Dassoff, PhD, Ira Levin, PhD, Janice Schreckengost, MA, AB, Stephen P. Stelzner, PhD, and B. Eileen Altman, PhD* (Vol. 6, No. 1, 1989). *"An invaluable compendium for the prevention practitioner, as well as the researcher, laying out the essentials for developing effective prevention programs in the community. . . . This is a book which should be in the prevention practitioner's library, to read, re-read, and ponder." (The Community Psychologist)*

Prevention: Toward a Multidisciplinary Approach, edited by Leonard A. Jason, PhD, Robert D. Felner, PhD, John N. Moritsugu, PhD, and Robert E. Hess, PhD* (Vol. 5, No. 2, 1987). *"Will not only be of intellectual value to the professional but also to students in courses aimed at presenting a refreshingly comprehensive picture of the conceptual and practical relationships between community and prevention." (Seymour B. Sarason, Associate Professor of Psychology, Yale University)*

Prevention and Health: Directions for Policy and Practice, edited by Alfred H. Katz, PhD, Jared A. Hermalin, PhD, and Robert E. Hess, PhD* (Vol. 5, No. 1, 1987). *Read about the most current efforts being undertaken to promote better health.*

The Ecology of Prevention: Illustrating Mental Health Consultation, edited by James G. Kelly, PhD, and Robert E. Hess, PhD* (Vol. 4, No. 3/4, 1987). *"Will provide the consultant with a very useful framework and the student with an appreciation for the time and commitment necessary to bring about lasting changes of a preventive nature." (The Community Psychologist)*

Monographs "Separates" list continued at the back

Indexing, Abstracting & Website/Internet Coverage

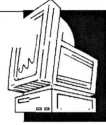

This section provides you with a list of major indexing & abstracting services and other tools for bibliographic access. That is to say, each service began covering this periodical during the year noted in the right column. Most Websites which are listed below have indicated that they will either post, disseminate, compile, archive, cite or alert their own Website users with research-based content from this work. (This list is as current as the copyright date of this publication.)

Abstracting, Website/Indexing Coverage . . . . Year When Coverage Began

- *Behavioral Medicine Abstracts* **1996**

- *CAB ABSTRACTS c/o CAB International/CAB ACCESS . . . .*
  available in print, diskettes updated weekly, and on
  INTERNET. Providing full bibliographic listings, author
  affiliation, augmented keyword searching.
  <http://www.cabi.org/> **2004**

- *CINAHL (Cumulative Index to Nursing & Allied Health*
  Literature), in print, EBSCO, and SilverPlatter, Data-Star,
  and PaperChase. (Support materials include Subject
  Heading List, Database Search Guide, and instructional
  video). <http://www.cinahl.com> **2003**

- *Educational Research Abstracts (ERA) (online database)*
  <http://www.tandf.co.uk/era>. **2002**

- *EMBASE/Excerpta Medica Secondary Publishing Division.*
  Included in newsletters, review journals, major reference works,
  magazines & abstract journals <http://www.elsevier.nl> **1996**

- *EMBASE.com (The Power of EMBASE + MEDLINE Combined)*
  <http://www.embase.com> **1996**

(continued)

(continued)

*Special Bibliographic Notes related to special journal issues
(separates) and indexing/abstracting:*

- indexing/abstracting services in this list will also cover material in any "separate" that is co-published simultaneously with Haworth's special thematic journal issue or DocuSerial. Indexing/abstracting usually covers material at the article/chapter level.
- monographic co-editions are intended for either non-subscribers or libraries which intend to purchase a second copy for their circulating collections.
- monographic co-editions are reported to all jobbers/wholesalers/approval plans. The source journal is listed as the "series" to assist the prevention of duplicate purchasing in the same manner utilized for books-in-series.
- to facilitate user/access services all indexing/abstracting services are encouraged to utilize the co-indexing entry note indicated at the bottom of the first page of each article/chapter/contribution.
- this is intended to assist a library user of any reference tool (whether print, electronic, online, or CD-ROM) to locate the monographic version if the library has purchased this version but not a subscription to the source journal.
- individual articles/chapters in any Haworth publication are also available through the Haworth Document Delivery Service (HDDS).

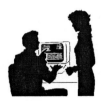

ABOUT THE EDITOR

Steven Godin, PhD, MPH, CHES, received his BA Degree in Social-Personality Psychology from the California State University, Fullerton, CA in 1980. He received his MS Degree in Community Psychology in 1983 and his PhD in Clinical-Community Psychology in 1989 from the Illinois Institute of Technology, Chicago, Illinois. Dr. Godin has been a Certified Health Education Specialist (CHES) since 1991. He has been a licensed psychologist in New Jersey since 1992. Dr. Godin completed a post-doctorate Masters in Public Health in 1994 from the joint program offered at the University of Medicine and Dentistry of New Jersey and the Edward Bloustein School of Planning and Public Policy at Rutgers University. Dr. Godin is a member of the American Psychological Association, Society for Prevention Research, and the American Public Health Association.

Dr. Godin is a Professor and Coordinator of the Community Health Education Undergraduate Program at East Stroudsburg University (ESU). He is a member of the graduate public health faculty at ESU teaching "computer applications," "evaluation research," and "public health measurement science" for the CEPH accredited MPH program. He also serves as a Clinical Professor and core faculty member within the APA approved PsyD doctorate program in Clinical Psychology at the Philadelphia College of Osteopathic Medicine (PCOM) located in Philadelphia. At PCOM, he teaches experimental design, graduate statistics sequence, "program planning and evaluation in community mental health," and is a chairperson for a number of PsyD dissertations.

In 1997, Dr. Godin started his own consulting firm–"Skylands Public & Behavioral Health Consulting" where he and his staff provide technical assistance to hospitals, agencies, pharmaceuticals, and state departments of health in the development and evaluation of Internet-based health promotion and health behavior change programs. Presently, he is working on the development and evaluation of a number of Internet-based prevention projects. Some of these include: (1) The development of an Internet-based

"Diabetes Disease Management Program" that includes educational modules on foot care; (2) The development of an Internet-based "Cancer Community Toolbox" to build local capacity to improve cancer health literacy, early detection and screening for cancer, for residents of New Jersey and Pennsylvania; and (3) Evaluating the impact of digital intake technologies on consumers' treatment adherence in disease management.

Over the past 15 years (1990-04), Dr. Godin has received over $3 million in grants and contracts to conduct prevention programs and program evaluation research. Dr. Godin is the author/co-author of over 40 publications and technical/research reports and has made over 100 professional presentations at international, national, regional and state conferences. He has also given many local public presentations including a number of appearances on radio and television.

Dr. Godin resides with his wife Deirdre, and children Lindsay (age 12) and Ryan (age 8) in Lebanon, New Jersey. Being raised in southern California, he remains fixated on visiting the beach, is a diehard sports fan, and takes his golf game very seriously.

Technology Applications in Prevention

CONTENTS

Technology Applications in Prevention: An Introduction

Steven Godin

East Stroudsburg University

PREDISPOSING FACTORS: THE U.S. HEALTH CARE SYSTEM

Presently, the health care industry is the number two employer of the United States workforce. In 2001, Americans spent $1.4 trillion on health care services, which was approximately 14% of the gross domestic product (GDP) for the country. Cost containment strategies (i.e., managed care) in the 1990s held health care spending constant; however, in the last three years, the country has witnessed significant inflationary pressures in health care. Annually, costs of providing health services are rising between 8% to 12%, creating significant economic pressures on business and industry. As a result of these increases, in 2000 approximately 20% of employers changed their health insurance plans as a cost savings strategy. Many of these new plans have reduced breadth of coverage or have increased employee deductibles (see Ferman, 2003; McCarthy, 2003; Oberlander, 2003). Furthermore, many companies are curtailing preventive health care benefits (i.e., wellness exams) or are scaling back on outpatient mental health coverage to reduce health insurance costs even though the outcomes literature has demonstrated these services actually save money in the long-term.

[Haworth co-indexing entry note]: "Technology Applications in Prevention: An Introduction." Godin, Steven. Co-published simultaneously in *Journal of Prevention & Intervention in the Community* (The Haworth Press, Inc.) Vol. 29, No. 1/2, 2005, pp. 1-6; and: *Technology Applications in Prevention* (ed: Steven Godin) The Haworth Press, Inc., 2005, pp. 1-6. Single or multiple copies of this article are available for a fee from The Haworth Document Delivery Service [1-800-HAWORTH, 9:00 a.m. - 5:00 p.m. (EST). E-mail address: docdelivery@haworthpress.com].

http://www.haworthpress.com/web/JPIC
Digital Object Identifier: 10.1300/J005v29n01_01

1

Nonetheless, as the baby-boomer population continues to age, these rising costs in health and mental health are expected to continue. By 2010, health care costs are forecasted to approach 20% of the GDP in the United States. In the past, the United States has never had a history nor reputation for the primary prevention of social problems. In consequence, the country will continue its legacy for responding to a tertiary crisis by finally addressing the health care exigency. In turn, primary prevention and technological application of preventive interventions will lead the way in reducing health care costs.

ENVISIONING THE FUTURE

In the next decade, as employers and insurance companies scramble to provide affordable health care coverage, there will be an ever-increasing emphasis on cost effectiveness and accountability in health care practices. Cost containment of health care in the future will focus on "best practices" in prevention of disease, and cost effective strategies for tertiary services in the form of "disease management." The increased attention given to evidence-based medicine will show repeatedly (as preventionists have known for decades) that the modification of maladaptive behaviors that lead to disease and mental illness are the most cost effective. Furthermore, outcome studies will continue to provide evidence that management of health behaviors is equally effective, and, in some cases, more effective than costly pharmacological interventions. These findings will not be surprising since 70% of all disease states and health conditions have a behavioral etiology.

Concurrent with the cost containment struggle, federal and state funding agencies and a variety of philanthropic foundations will focus their educative efforts on consumer empowerment and skill building to prevent disease and mental illness. As the rising costs of health care creates an ever-increasing burden on the funding of primary prevention, the implementation of technological innovations and use of the Internet in delivering efficient and cost effective interventions will ultimately save the health care system. While the U.S. government will struggle to ensure parity in access to health care, it will succeed in its empowerment efforts to improve the nation's "health literacy." Through building consumers' health and mental health literacy (i.e., having knowledge and skills about maintaining healthy behaviors), a culture will develop where the public will be empowered to delay the onset of costly diseases, health conditions, and mental illness. The Internet will become one of the leading venues by which health literacy will be accomplished.

One technological tool to improve the nation's health literacy will be the use of the computer and the Internet. The cost of computers is now on par with the price of television sets, and the cost of Internet access continues to decline. While computer ownership and Internet adoption has begun to saturate the middle to high-income population, the highest percentage increase is now occurring within the $15,000/yr. and lower income brackets (Birru 7 Steinman, 2004; Shapiro & Rohde, 2000; U.S. Department of Commerce, 2004). According to the report published by the U.S. Department of Commerce (2004), about 55% of U.S. households in 2003 had access to the Internet, while only one-third of households with income less than $15,000 had access. However, in reviewing the data from this report, adoption of the Internet increases each year by about 3-5% in middle income and about 6-7% in low-income families. Thus, by 2010, it can be estimated that household Internet access in the U.S. will approach 75-90% for middle-income families, and approximately 70-80% for low-income households. While these figures are just estimates, clearly adoption of the Internet continues and presents a viable tool for preventionists to use in reaching a variety of target populations

CONTENTS OF THIS VOLUME

Technology Applications in Prevention provides nine manuscripts that offer a snapshot of the current state of the art approaches in applying technology to prevention and intervention. This volume starts out with a manuscript from Pokorny and his colleagues from DePaul University entitled "Efficient and Effective Uses of Technology in Community Research." I placed this article at the beginning of this volume because of its vision and importance in our continued efforts to empirically validate prevention and community-based intervention programs. Future prevention researchers and program evaluators will need to become more knowledgeable about electronic data collection, management, and analyses to keep costs low. The article is strong in its efforts to provide examples of how useful technology can be in providing efficient and cost effective approaches in conducting prevention research.

Next, Shull and Berkowitz from the University of Massachusetts Lowell provide a manuscript entitled "Community Building with Technology: The Development of Collaborative Community Technology Initiatives in a Mid-Size City." In the spirit of the University of Kansas "Community Toolbox" (see *ctb.lsi.ukans.edu*), Shull and Berkowitz provide an case example of how Websites could function as regional clearinghouses of useful information, as well as provide a convenient forum for agency staff to update their prevention skills.

The third manuscript entitled "Applying Web-Based Survey Design Standards" addresses a critical concern that many have in "e-data collection": Is the needs assessment and/or outcome data collected on the Web reliable? Crawford and his colleagues from MSIResearch and the University of Michigan provide detailed information about survey design and visual presentation interface with users completing Internet-based questionnaires. All too often, researchers upload traditional paper-pencil surveys onto a Website without considering the "human factors issues" involved in Web-based data collection. In order for technology tools to maximize the efficacy of prevention efforts, certain standards should be adhered to in Internet-based data collection.

From East Stroudsburg University, the fourth manuscript entitled "Assessing Quality Assurance of Self-Help Sites on the Internet" by Godin and Colleagues and the fifth manuscript entitled "The Quality of Spanish Health Information Websites: An Emerging Disparity" by Cardelle and Rodriguez address the lack of quality in mental health and health information presented on the World Wide Web. While accessing health information has been one of the primary reasons people use the Internet, the lack of comprehensive quality assurance standards is an impediment towards achieving consumer health literacy. Furthermore, as the authors mention, few Websites have evolved to harness the power of the Internet in creating theory-based behavior change interventions. To date, the majority of sites provide consumers with "old wine in newly bottled" print media on the Internet. Many Websites provide consumers with information (sometimes inaccurate) without providing opportunities for consumer interaction or assessing consumers' comprehension. For health literacy to be realized, preventionists need to apply the lessons learned in education over the last half-century and improve the methods for providing trustworthy, comprehensible health and mental health information.

In the sixth manuscript entitled "A Participatory Internet Initiative in an African American Neighborhood," Suarez-Balcazar from the University of Illinois at Chicago and her Chicago colleagues address the health disparity concerns regarding use of the Internet. At the time of this publication, the Internet will have come close to saturating the middle income marketplace. The fastest growth in the Internet adoption curve is now occurring within the low-income communities. Again, if health literacy is to occur within society, we need to empower those who are digitally divided, and improve access for all to the Internet. Furthermore, once the divided get online . . . we need to ensure that the material provided is culturally relevant and appropriate.

In the seventh manuscript entitled "Alcohol Abuse Prevention Among High-Risk Youth," Schinke and his colleagues at Columbia University provide a case example of a CD-ROM life-skills-based intervention to prevent alcohol abuse. Over the years, preventionists have neglected to tap into the "edutainment" ideology that interfaces video gaming with life skills for the prevention of maladaptive health behaviors. As the Internet continues to evolve, I envision Web bandwidth to improve to where "reality TV"-based role plays can be provided in real-time scenarios as youth (and adults) learn to apply effective life skills to tailored social situations in an effort to reduce specific risk behaviors.

As Web bandwidth improves, theory-based skill-building interventions such as "Constructing Better Futures via Video" authored by Dowrick from the University of Hawaii at Mano and his colleagues from the University of Alaska Anchorage may be a mainstay on the Internet. To date, technology applications in prevention have neglected to move beyond the superficial practice of health behavior change theories.

Last, if technological advances in prevention are to be realized, the prevention profession must recognize the viability of the Internet as an intervention tool. Brown and her colleagues from the University of South Florida and Hunter College author a manuscript entitled "General Characteristics of Internet Use Among Health Educators: Implications for the Professions" which provides innovators with some insights as to the barriers and supports for adopting the Internet as a prevention tool. If the Internet is to evolve as an apparatus for obtaining consumer health literacy and empowering consumers to achieve and maintain healthy behaviors, so too must technology training evolve within the prevention field.

REFERENCES

Birru M., Steinman, R.A. (2004). Online health information and low-literacy African Americans, *Journal of Medical Research, 6,* e26.

Ferman, J.H. (2003). The rising cost of healthcare: Cost increases drive healthcare to the top of the domestic policy agenda. *Healthcare Executive, 18,* 70-71.

McCarthy, M. (2003). US health-care system faces cost and insurance crises: Rising costs, growing numbers of uninsured, and quality gaps trouble world's most expensive health-care system. *Lancet, 362,* 375.

Oberlander, J. (2002). The US health care system: On a road to nowhere? *Canadian Medical Association Journal, 167,* 163-168.

Shapiro R., Rohde, G. (2000). Falling Throught the Net: Toward digital Inclusion. Washington, D.C.: National Telecommunications and Information Administration and Economics and Statistics Administration.

U.S. Department of Commerce (2004). A Nation Online: Entering the Broadband Age. U.S. Department of Commerce, Economics and Statistical Administration.

Efficient and Effective Uses of Technology in Community Research

Steven B. Pokorny
Leonard A. Jason
Dana M. Helzing
Joseph Sherk
P. Jacob Rebus

Charlotte Kunz
Olga Rabin-Belyaev
Aaron Ostergaard
Kathleen Mikulski
Peter Y. Ji

DePaul University

SUMMARY. This paper describes how a research team at DePaul University is applying recent advances in technology to facilitate the implementation of a large-scale, community research project. The application of technology by members of the social sciences has often focused on advances in computational technologies to provide faster and more sophisticated ways to analyze data. However, there is less documentation of how technology can provide opportunities to improve the way scientists conduct community research. Social and community interventions can profit from technological innovations to alleviate difficulties in collecting, pro-

Address correspondence to: Steven B. Pokorny, PhD, Director, Youth Tobacco Access Project, DePaul University, Center for Community Research, 990 West Fullerton Avenue, Suite 3100, Chicago, IL 60614.

For more information about the authors' project activities, please visit their Website (http://condor. depaul.edu/~ljason/smoking) or see their other papers listed in the reference section.

The authors appreciate the support provided by the Robert Wood Johnson Foundation Substance Abuse Policy Research Program and the National Cancer Institute.

[Haworth co-indexing entry note]: "Efficient and Effective Uses of Technology in Community Research." Pokorny, Steven B. et al. Co-published simultaneously in *Journal of Prevention & Intervention in the Community* (The Haworth Press, Inc.) Vol. 29, No. 1/2, 2005, pp. 7-27; and: *Technology Applications in Prevention* (ed: Steven Godin) The Haworth Press, Inc., 2005, pp. 7-27. Single or multiple copies of this article are available for a fee from The Haworth Document Delivery Service [1-800-HAWORTH, 9:00 a.m. - 5:00 p.m. (EST). E-mail address: docdelivery@haworthpress.com].

http://www.haworthpress.com/web/JPIC
Digital Object Identifier: 10.1300/J005v29n01_02

cessing, managing, archiving, and sharing data. If researchers within the field of community psychology become more knowledgeable and competent in the use of technology, larger and more complex projects can be implemented in an efficient and effective manner. *[Article copies available for a fee from The Haworth Document Delivery Service: 1-800-HAWORTH. E-mail address: <docdelivery@haworthpress.com> Website: <http://www. HaworthPress.com> © 2005 by The Haworth Press, Inc. All rights reserved.]*

KEYWORDS. Community research, technology, tobacco, prevention, evolution

Society is becoming increasingly competent at using sophisticated technology. For example, advances in telecommunication technology improved people's ability to communicate with others, as well as changed the nature of these communications. In the private sector, many businesses capitalized on technological advances to increase productivity and to decrease costs. The social sciences used advances in computational technologies to provide faster and more sophisticated ways to analyze data. However, there are few examples of how advances in technology provide opportunities to improve the way community psychologists conduct research.

This paper describes how a research team at DePaul University is applying recent advances in technology to conduct a large-scale, multi-year, community research project. The introduction of technological innovations into the field of community research helped to alleviate some of the difficulties in collecting, processing, managing, archiving, and sharing data. The Youth Tobacco Access Project at DePaul University was aided by the use of specific technologies, and we highlight how the use of these innovations assisted this project with overcoming common research hurdles.

PROJECT OVERVIEW

The Youth Tobacco Access Project is a social-policy intervention that aims to reduce youth tobacco use through the enforcement of local tobacco-control laws (Jason & Pokorny, 2002; Jason, Pokorny, & Schoeny, 2003). The current project is funded by a grant from the National Cancer Institute (NCI). From 1999 to 2001, the Robert Wood Johnson Foundation funded a pilot study during which all assessment measures were developed and tested. Over a five-year period, the current NCI project will systematically examine the impact of tobacco-control laws on the prevalence of smoking and other tobacco use among seventh through twelfth grade students in 24 communities. Participating communities were randomly assigned into two groups. The first group enforces laws prohibiting the sale of tobacco to minors. The second group enforces laws prohibiting the sale of tobacco to minors and laws that prohibit possession of tobacco by minors.

Our research team collects two main types of outcome data in the participating communities. The first major data source is an annual student survey, which assesses the prevalence of tobacco use among youth in the participating communities. The survey is administered to the seventh through twelfth grade students in each community. Students typically complete the survey in 20 to 25 minutes. This survey is an eight-page document consisting of 73 questions. Of these questions, 54 have multiple-choice responses (i.e., with a range of 3-12 choices), 16 have dichotomous choice responses, and 3 have a combination of multiple-choice and fill-in-the-blank responses. A total of 11,234 students completed the survey in the first wave of data collection.

The second major data source is an annual assessment of the rate of illegal tobacco sales to minors in each community. This assessment measures the extent that minors have access to retail sources of tobacco. All tobacco retailers in each community are assessed through a procedure whereby a 15- or 16-year-old youth enters the establishment and attempts to purchase cigarettes. Following this tobacco purchase attempt, the youth reports information about the outcome and other relevant details (e.g., presence of signs about the tobacco sales law, self-service displays, promotions, etc.) to a member of the research team who completes a one-page data form. The data form consists of 31 questions, of which 20 are multiple choice type questions and 11 are fill-in-the-blank type questions. A total of 542 retailers were assessed in the first wave of data collection.

In addition, our research team collects information on other relevant characteristics of the communities and schools. Specifically, we collect data on community readiness for this type of intervention (Engstrom, Jason, Townsend, Pokorny, & Curie, 2002), comprehensiveness of local tobacco-control laws (Pokorny, Townsend, Jason, Lautenschlager, & Smith, 2002), quality of school-based tobacco prevention programs (Townsend, Pokorny, Jason, Curie, & Schoeny, 2002), factors related to illegal tobacco sales to minors (Curie, Pokorny, Jason, Schoeny, & Townsend, 2002), and potential risks for minors participating in tobacco purchase attempts (Ji, Pokorny, Blaszkowski, Jason, & Rabin-Belyaev, 2002). Together, these data provide a comprehensive view of the impact of the intervention as well as other factors related to youth tobacco use.

DATA COLLECTION

The success of any research endeavor depends, in part, on collecting accurate and reliable information. Frequently, community psychologists want to collect data about the broader social settings in which they work. Collecting this type of information can be challenging for large, multi-community studies. Our research team uses the Internet and a computer-aided mapping program to facilitate data collection with the 24 participating communities.

The Internet

A significant component of the Youth Tobacco Access Project is the compilation of a variety of data concerning the towns, schools, and police departments that participate in the study. Collecting this type of information can be a time-consuming process, requiring extensive resources spent in a library or a town record hall. However, the Internet is changing the manner in which scientists collect information. It makes the task of collecting data more efficient and less burdensome. The Internet has been referred to as "a powerful resource for research, providing limitless access to information" (Lindsay, 2000). As described below, our research team uses the Internet for a number of data collection tasks.

Advantages of Using the Internet. The Internet plays a critical role, as town informant, for the project. Our research team is able to obtain valuable information about a community quickly. The majority of participating towns have government-run Web sites. According to a poll conducted by the National League of Cities, 89 percent of cities in the U.S. have their own Web site (Perry, 2000). These Web sites often provide the names and addresses of important town officials, thus providing important contact information. Our research team also relies on the Internet to provide detailed demographic information about a town. For example, our research team needs to obtain information about the total population, the population under 18 years of age, ethnic composition, and median income for each community. This information is easily accessible to the public via the Internet. Census data on every community in the United States can also be obtained from the U.S. Census Bureau government Web page (U.S. Census Bureau, 2000).

Another phase of the project involves surveying students from one junior high and one high school in each town. Our research team collects a variety of information about the composition and performance of each participating school to control for possible school effects on the outcome variables. These demographic and performance data can be found on the Internet via the Illinois State Board of Education Web page (Illinois State Board of Education, 2001). This Web site, among other information, provides each Illinois School's Report Card. The School Report Card provides such pertinent information as racial/ethnic composition, attendance, mobility, total enrollment, proportion of low-income students, and academic performance. Internet access to this information saves a significant amount of time and effort.

In addition, our research team also uses the Internet to collect logistical information. This is accomplished through the use of directory and mapping services provided on the Internet. The Internet provides comprehensive directions to each location, eliminating the need for developing routes manually. The Internet Yellow Pages Directory provides names and addresses of tobacco vendors, police departments, and schools. This Internet-provided service also permits our research team to locate and to identify tobacco vendors in towns that do have a list of tobacco retailers because of local tobacco-license law. A complete list of all potential tobacco retailers (e.g., gas stations, restaurants, convenience stores, liquor stores, bars, and hotels) within a town is created through a directory search. Our research team then contacts each of these businesses by phone to determine if the merchant sells any tobacco products. The Internet also helps our research team maintain a paperless office. Given the scope and magnitude of this study, without access to the Internet, it would be necessary to maintain and organize 24 different phone directories, one for each participating community.

Disadvantages of Using the Internet. Despite the numerous advantages offered by the Internet, there are some limitations, including missing, outdated, or invalid information. Some efforts to collect town information fail because a participating town may have either an inadequate or nonexistent Web site. Costs associated with creating and maintaining a Web site may prevent some communities from taking advantage of this technology. According to one expert, Internet Web sites can "range from several hundred dollars for a simple site consisting of a few pages to a half million dollars or more for advanced sites" (Goldsborough, 2001). The process of creating and maintaining a Web site is also quite arduous. Once the site is created, it must be submitted to a host, given a domain name, submitted to a Web search service, and then continually updated. Lack of resources may also inhibit the implementation of a Web site. Strover (2001) suggests that remote or rural areas may not have a sufficient telecommunications infrastructure to support adequate connection to the Internet. The author further suggests that this may be due in part to the insufficient governmental funding for small communities to develop such infrastructure.

Another limitation of Internet-based information is that it can be unreliable or out-of-date. On more than one occasion, our research team acquired the name of a town official from the Internet only to learn that the official's term ended the previous year. Another example of this problem occurred when our research team obtained inaccurate directions to a participating school.

Mapping Vendors

Mapping the locations of tobacco vendors within a town presents a large and time-consuming task for our research team. This is a necessary step in the preparation for the tobacco purchase attempts, which assess the rate of illegal tobacco sales to minors. Our research team must drive a minor to every tobacco vendor within each town in order to complete the assessment. However, our research team typically does not know each town well enough to navigate from vendor to vendor without a well-constructed map. The list of local tobacco vendors must be transformed into a working map. Initially, our research team completed this task manually. A member of our research team obtained a map of the town and used an Internet program, which required the vendor's address, to produce a small map of the location. Finally, each of these small maps was used to transfer the exact location to the town map. However, this process was time-consuming and labor intensive. New technology based on a geographic information system is a computer-aided mapping program that provides a more efficient way to complete this task.

Advantages of Using Geographic Information Systems. BusinessMAP PRO (Environmental Systems Research Institute [ESRI], 1996) is a computer-aided mapping program that permits the user to represent various types of information geographically. Using this program, a member of the research team can quickly map the locations of each tobacco retailer in a community. First, a member of the research team enters the address for each tobacco vendor in a participating town into a single spreadsheet. That spreadsheet is then linked to the mapping program, which plots the points within each town. The program allows our research team to choose the detail with which the map is created (i.e., streets, major highways, town names, county lines, etc.). The mapping program contains all of the maps of the participating towns and only requires the addresses of the vendors to prepare the maps. The efficiency achieved by this technology is impressive: A town of one hundred vendors took an entire eight-hour workday to map-out manually. In contrast, when using the mapping program for the same town, it only took a total of thirty minutes to enter the addresses of the vendors, create the map, and verify that all addresses were plotted correctly. The latest version of this software has several new features that could be useful to community psychologists. BusinessMAP III has updated geographic information including zip codes; provides 500 Census 2000 demographic variables down to the census tract level; gives address-to-address and optimized routing information; and can create maps based on specific geographical information like counties, zip codes, or census tracts (ESRI, 2002). These new features can give community psychologists a new way to visualize communities.

Disadvantages of Using Geographic Information Systems. There are a few limitations of relying on geographic information systems. Many communities in the U.S. are expanding, and information in the program about streets and roads in a community can become outdated. Our research team experienced several instances in which the program would not recognize the name of a street. In addition, the program is not 100 percent accurate in mapping the location of addresses. During our first wave of data collection, the program incorrectly mapped the locations of one percent of the retailers. These errors cost the research team additional time and energy trying to find the retailers while in the field.

DATA PROCESSING

Data processing is perhaps one of the most labor-intensive tasks within a research project. The amount of data collected and the necessity that it be processed in a timely manner can be an enormous drain on project resources. Many researchers in the field of community psychology use paper and pencil surveys to collect information from participants. Typically, these surveys are hand scored and then manually entered into a computer for analysis. Our research team has addressed this challenge by automating the data processing tasks with a computer-based information capture system.

Information Capture System

TELEform is a computer-based information capture system that permits the user to design data collection forms, scan the data into the computer, verify inaccurate responses, and export the data to a statisical software program (Cardiff Software Inc., 1991). Data collection forms are printed on a high-volume printer to produce quality copies that can be easily scanned. After data collection, a high-volume scanner inputs the data to a computer. Finally, an optical recognition program verifies the accuracy of the data and exports the data in a variety of formats supported by statistical software programs. Automating data processing tasks enables the project to operate with a small staff and limited resources, yet maintain efficiency in the processing of field data.

Advantages of Using Information Capture Systems. TELEform has numerous capabilities that aid in the data collection, processing, and management tasks. Our research team is able to create personalized data forms that are designed to be user friendly and are organized for efficient data collection. This technology offers an improvement over generic scan-type forms that are sometimes used when collecting survey data. The custom forms reduce the chance for response error because the question and response set appear together rather than off to the side or on a separate form, making it less likely for survey participants to miscode answer sheets.

The data forms are scanned into a computer, at which time the software sorts the data, codes recognizable entries, and flags unrecognizable data. Our research team is able to view a digital image of the actual form that was scanned and manually verify only those items that have been flagged by the program as unrecognizable. Additionally, TELEform allows the user to set a desired confidence interval at which it screens the data, and this results in fewer errors than when data are manually entered. The verified data are exported, in a format that is compatible with a variety of software applications, to a statistical program for analysis.

It would take considerable time and staff resources to manually enter thousands of student surveys and hundreds of data forms each year. Our research team could not perform research on the scale that it does without this sophisticated information capture system software. The following case study illustrates the efficiency with which data are processed. Approximately 1,200 students were surveyed in a town during a single school day. Preparation of these surveys for scanning (i.e., removing staples and straightening bent corners on forms) took two hours. Scanning the surveys took two hours and 40 minutes. The software sorted, organized, and coded the scanned images overnight. The following day, one member of the research team verified the flagged items (i.e., unclear responses) in two hours and 30 minutes. The data, with all variable labels and value labels, were automatically exported by the application into a format ready to use by the statistical software program. Our research team completed the analyses in 30 minutes and wrote the school's report in two hours. All totaled, less than 10 hours of staff time was required for complete processing and analysis of this large data set.

Jorgensen and Karlsmose (1998) conducted a study that measured the efficiency and effectiveness of this information capture system. These authors estimated that data processing time using this technology took one-third to one-half less time than manual data-entry and that wage expenses were reduced by one-quarter to one-third when using this application.

Community-based research frequently involves time-sensitive data, which is useful only when it is processed and analyzed quickly so that it can be shared with the community. Our research team faces such time-related concerns when students graduate from one school and move to another school in the community. If our research team were unable to report findings prior to such a move, the data they collected would be less relevant to the participating school. This technology makes it possible for the research team to complete all the steps from data collection to community feedback in less than one month's time.

In addition, the ability to give timely feedback to participants reinforces the community's involvement in the study. A common complaint heard by our research team during the recruitment of communities is that they have felt unappreciated and uninformed by other researchers. This was often a result of receiving little or no feedback regarding the results of the study. A research team's ability to provide thorough, prompt feedback meets participants' information needs and reinforces their decision to participate. Dissemination of research findings is a key step in the model for community involvement proposed by Bracht and Kingsbury (1990). These authors conclude that maintaining high visibility through communication of the findings is critical for sustaining community involvement.

Disadvantages of Using Information Capture Systems. Despite the advantages, there are some limitations to using this type of technology in research. While in the long term technology can save time, a considerable amount of time also needs to be invested initially to set up the technology for the specific project, to train staff in how to use the technology, and to maintain the technology so that it remains useful. For this reason, the time invested in setup, training, and maintenance must be less than the time saved for the technology to be efficient. In the case of this information capture system, it only becomes cost-effective when large quantities of data forms are being processed (Jorgensen & Karlsmose, 1998). In addition, sophisticated technology may be more prone to develop problems. Allowing a project to become too dependent on technology can compromise an entire project if the technology is not functioning properly. When technological problems occur, the staff resources can be diverted from the primary research objectives.

DATA MANAGEMENT

Collection and processing of data are critical aspects of the research process. However, multi-year projects also require effective management of the collected information. Over the course of the current five-year study, our project requires the collection of records and contact information for each of the 24 towns, including the police department, the high school, and the junior high school. In addition, our research team has already accumulated over 500 pieces of reference material that is relevant to our work. Managing this amount of information including updates and reports can be a challenging task. Our research team meets this challenge by using relational database software and reference management software.

Relational Database Software

One way to manage the large amount of information generated by a research project is to create a number of spreadsheets, each comprised of numerous cells. However, this process would be both time-consuming and inefficient. For example, a large number of spreadsheets with unique names would be difficult to navigate when looking for specific information. Also, the vast amount of information could result in excessively large spreadsheets that make it difficult to view specific information without either reducing the size of the entire spreadsheet or removing unnecessary cells. For example, if all of the school information were stored in a single spreadsheet, it would be hard to quickly identify the 12 participating schools that required Spanish versions of the survey material. When the spreadsheet is opened, the information for all of the participating schools would appear and even the names of the 24 towns alone would not fit onto the screen. Locating the specific information would require scrolling up and down through the spreadsheet. In addition, information frequently needs to be repeated across spreadsheets (e.g., town name), which creates unnecessary overlap. Our research team solved this problem through the use of relational database software. A relational database stores all its data inside tables (i.e., spreadsheets) and all operations on data are done on the tables themselves or produce another table as the result.

Advantages of Using Relational Database Software. Technology provided by relational database software (e.g., Microsoft Access) can simplify the management of large amounts of information. The main advantage of relational database software is its ability to combine many sources of information into one system. Basically, a relational database links numerous spreadsheets with a common variable, which eliminates the need to duplicate information. Despite the complexity of the data, the operation of the program is quite simple. The expertise required to design and create the database depends on the complexity of the information that will be managed. A member of the research team can create a simple database by answering a series of easy questions, prompted by the program, to get a finished application with switchboards, data-entry screen, and report features. Occasionally, a technical expert will be needed to design a database containing complex information. For example, the current project requires management of town information (e.g., demographics, primary contacts, local tobacco merchants, etc.), police information (enforcement activity, primary contacts, local tobacco-control policies, etc.), and school information (demographics, primary contacts, school performance, etc.).

Relational database programs include features to facilitate data entry and data access. Some of these features ensure that only the specific type of information that belongs in a table or cell can be entered. For example, the program would not permit the letter "a" to be entered into a field designated for numeric information. This feature helps to maintain the integrity of the data in the database. In this respect, data entry is no more complex than that of a simple spreadsheet application. Access to data is also more efficient because the information is linked directly or indirectly to different spreadsheets. For example, the amount of information about different schools and police departments is so large that it is usually entered into separate spreadsheets. In order to access information about a town, including its police department, both the high school and a junior high, and any other information stored under a specific town, three or more spreadsheets may need to be opened to get the required information. To access the same type of information from a relational database, a query (i.e., request for a report) would be used to obtain only the desired information about that town. The problem presented in the earlier example of identifying schools that require survey materials in Spanish could also be solved by a query. The result of the query would produce a list of schools by type of survey material required. As illustrated by these examples, relational database software can provide access to large amounts of information in a faster and more efficient way.

Disadvantages of Using Relational Database Software. A major limitation to this type of technology is that a high level of expertise may be required to design, create, and maintain a database comprised of complex information. For example, the current project requires management of information about schools within towns as well as students within schools over a period of five years. For example, the longitudinal design requires our research team to track parent consent status for each student from year to year and across the transition from middle school to high school. This level of complexity necessitated hiring a consultant to aid with the design and creation of the database.

Reference Management Software

Large-scale, multi-year research projects are also faced with the task of managing reference material. Like many researchers who develop a program of research in an area, our research team has hard copy files of over 500 pieces of reference material. The challenge is to keep track of this amount of material and make it readily accessible by topic to members of the research team. Our research team uses a reference management program to accomplish this task.

Advantages of Using Reference Management Software. Specialized reference management software like Biblioscape (CG Information, 1997) is available and allows researchers to manage a large quantity of material in an organized and efficient way. These types of programs help researchers organize free-form information, conduct research online, and format papers. Biblioscape allows our research team to efficiently manage numerous reference books, articles, and journals in a common database that are accumulated during the course of the project.

The program sorts information into electronic folders and permits the user to categorize each article with keywords pertaining to the article's content, making it easier to locate references. References can be located through a search by keywords, publication year, author, or name of a journal. This feature gives our research team quick access to all project references on a given topic without requiring a member of the research team to search through hard copies in the project's archive. Conducting literature searches online is also more efficient. Bibliographic material that is readily available on the Web can be directly captured into the database through a built-in Web browser. This software program also incorporates Microsoft Word and WordPerfect to help format citations for manuscripts. This feature allows our research team to select from a variety of citation and bibliography formats to meet publisher requirements.

Biblioscape's ability to organize free-form information is an important asset for our research team. The advantage of a project-specific database is that it allows for fast retrieval of relevant documents. For example, a member of our research team enters a keyword, publication year, author, or journal title and gains efficient access to all of the relevant reference material in our files. Although this software needs to be updated manually, it is a much less time-consuming process than searching in a more general database or having to look through hard copies of articles. The organizational and time-saving benefits that reference management software provides are well worth the minimal effort it takes to maintain the system.

Disadvantages of Using Reference Management Software. The major limitation of this technology is that the software license only permits installation and use on a single computer. Consequently, the information is not readily accessible to everyone on the research team. This limitation also requires papers to be written on that computer to take advantage of the feature for auto formatting citations.

DATA ARCHIVING

Under the General Guidelines of the American Psychological Association (APA), raw data must be retained by the researcher for a minimum of three years after completion of the project, pending federal, state, and local laws (APA, 1993). The guidelines also state that all data with identifying information must be kept in a secure place to ensure the confidentiality of the persons involved. In the current NCI project, approximately 20,000 eight-page student surveys, 40,000 consent forms, and approximately 840 one-page tobacco purchase attempt data forms are collected each year. The storage issues are complicated because the consent forms need to be kept in a locked storage unit or a locked room. Our research team addressed this challenge by using digital imaging technology.

Digital Imaging

Data archiving problems were partially resolved in 2001 when the Institutional Review Board (IRB) at DePaul University decided to allow the storage of the student survey and tobacco purchase attempt data in digital form. As described earlier, these data were already scanned into the computer with the information capture system. The result of this process was the creation of image files (i.e., .tiff files), each representing a digital image of a page from the completed student surveys and data collection forms. The research team burned these image files onto data compact disks (CDs) for storage.

Advantages of Using Digital Imaging. The storage capacity of a data CD is about 30,000 one-page data forms. That capacity is increased when the files are compressed. The amount of space taken up by nearly sixty boxes holding 5,000 sheets each is condensed down to 10 CDs that can be easily locked in a drawer. The digital images that are stored on the CDs are exact copies of the hard data, and are easily accessed when properly labeled. Each CD data set is labeled for year, town, school, and vendor. All data, including the reports for participating schools and police departments, are saved onto CDs for storage. After digitally archiving the data, all hard copies are destroyed in mass quantity by a paper shredding company that provides verification of destruction. This is a necessary step to insure the confidentiality of the individuals involved in the research project. The ability to store data in this manner allows project space to be used more efficiently, creating more room for our research team and project equipment.

Digital storage of this information will reduce the amount of hard data that is being stored at the project facilities. However, obtaining permission for the digital storage of consent forms was more complicated. These forms constitute legal documents, and the ability to store these forms in digital format is controversial. The APA does not have existing guidelines for the electronic storage of these types of documents. One concern is the ability of the documents to be tampered with or changed when they are in a digital form. Storage of these documents in hard copy form creates a substantially smaller problem than storing the other types of data. However, in the pilot study, thousands of one-page consent forms were collected. This resulted in seven boxes of documents that required secure storage. In the current project, the numbers are estimated to reach approximately 40,000 consent forms a year. At a minimum, this would result in approximately 32 boxes of documents that will require secure storage by the end of the project.

A solution to this problem was found in recent state and federal legislation regarding the validity of electronic signatures. The E-Sign Act passed by Congress on June 30, 2000, confirmed that electronic signatures "may not be denied legal effect, validity, or enforceability solely because it is in electronic form" (Cohen, 2001). Specifically, E-Sign has record retention provisions that endorse the validity of documents converted from hard copy form into digital form (Wittie & Winn, 2000). Moreover, the E-Sign provisions allow for documents to be converted from one digital format to another, such as the transfer of image files from a computer hard drive onto CDs for storage. This provision includes updating documents to a new format that ensures future accessibility, as original storage formats become outdated. After consideration of the E-Sign Act and consultation with IRBs at other universities, the DePaul University IRB agreed to permit the storage of consent forms in a digital format. This procedure will enable the project to store all of the pilot and current project's consent forms in a single locked file cabinet in contrast to the approximately 39 boxes of hard copies of these documents.

Disadvantages of Using Digital Imaging. The major limitation of using digital imaging technology for data storage is the additional staff resources required to scan the documents to get them into digital format. As described earlier, scanning the surveys and data collection forms was completed as part of our data processing task, but scanning the parent consent forms required additional staff resources. In addition, the documents to be scanned must be in good condition for the process to be efficient, which may require further preparation. For example, some of the parent consent forms were in poor condition (e.g., torn corners, folds, and wrinkles) and had to be photocopied before they could be scanned.

DATA SHARING

An important way that technology benefits researchers is by allowing a faster and more efficient means to conduct research and share that information. Our research team has taken advantage of such innovations as a shared computer network to greatly improve the efficiency of their work. In the same way that technology has aided in the research process, it has also improved the ability to communicate findings from the project to surrounding communities and other interested individuals. Through the use of the Internet, individuals are able to share information with millions of people throughout the world (Nazarali-Stranieri, 2000). Our research team utilizes a computer network, electronic mail, Web pages, and faxes to communicate up-to-date information to those inside and outside of the project in a fast, efficient manner.

Computer Network

The computer network used by our research team has become an indispensable aid to communication within the project. All members of the project have access to a shared network drive, which links all of the projects computers to a common intranet. This gives members of our research team the ability to access all files concerning the project from his/her own personal computer. The shared network allows multiple individuals on separate computers to pool all of their work into one common source.

Advantages of Using a Computer Network. Computer network technology allows team members to work collaboratively to update and maintain project files. This system also increases the speed and efficiency in which our research team is able to retrieve data. All of the data, ranging from interview data to reports from previous years, are stored digitally on the network. Our research team is able to find information quickly and finish the tasks on the project instead of searching through large files of paper documents. In addition, the shared network facilitates the revision of documents because a hard copy is not necessary in order to edit or comment on the work of other team members. Due to the shared access to the files, feedback can be given almost immediately and appropriate changes can be made. For example, a feature in the word-processing software allows our research team to track the editing process when writing reports to disseminate to schools and police departments in participating communities. This feature highlights revisions and updates and permits the original author to view the changes made and decide whether to accept or reject them. This provides an efficient and productive method for exchanging feedback and completing the reports.

Disadvantages of Using a Computer Network. Despite the advantages of a shared network, there are also limitations that should be considered. Since the information is stored on the network, progress on the project is stalled when the network is down because the information is not accessible. Another disadvantage of the shared network is when multiple users are working on the same file, only one person is able to make changes and save the file. The other users can access the file as "read only," which enables them to view the document, but not make any changes. While this sounds inconvenient, it is rare that two members of the research team need to revise a document simultaneously. These disadvantages can present inconveniences to our research team at times.

Electronic Mail and Web Sites

Connections from the shared network to the Internet and electronic mail (e-mail) providers help to promote the transfer of information and the findings of the study to the community at large. E-mail and Web sites are widely accepted forms of communication for a large portion of the population. E-mail communication systems use a variety of software to create and deliver messages over the Internet. Web sites on the Internet provide a vast amount of resource information, and specific types of information can be located by using software-based search engines.

Advantages of Using E-Mail and Web Sites. Communicating information and research findings helps to inform and educate members of a community, which in turn has an empowering effect on the participants' desire for positive social change (Samuel, 2000). Project participants include police officers and school administrators who are sometimes difficult to contact by phone because they are often away from their office. E-mail provides an effective communication tool for such individuals because the message remains in a mailbox until the individual can respond. This communication medium also allows our research team to send documents as attachments. Consequently, participants can have immediate access to necessary documents in digital form. For example, our research team sends a template of a letter of support to each of the participating principals. The principals modify the letter as needed and print the final document on the schools' stationery. This process facilitates collaboration with the principals and reduces the amount of time and effort required.

Our research team also developed a Web site for the project to provide participants and others access to information about the project (http://condor.depaul.edu/~ljason/smoking). Data from previous studies, relevant publications, and measures are made available through this Web site. Maintaining a Web site provides credibility to the research and helps to inform community members about the goals of the project.

The Web site is also an efficient way for other researchers and community members to learn about tobacco prevention and our project.

Disadvantages of Using E-Mail and Web Sites. A major limitation of using e-mail technology as a communication mode is the incompatibility of different software platforms. For example, text within the main body of the message usually gets through fine, but frequently attached documents cannot be read. Another limitation with e-mail is that some people are afraid to use it because computer viruses are frequently transmitted to computers through e-mail messages. The major limitation of using a Web site as a communication mode is the amount of resources required to design and maintain the Web site. Some general knowledge about the programming language HTML is usually required to develop an interesting Web site, and one must devote some time on a regular basis to keep the information up to date.

CONCLUSION

Technology offers community researchers many advantages when conducting large-scale projects. As an example, the Internet provides a wealth of information that can aid data collection tasks. In this paper, we have shown how the Internet can be utilized to collect a variety of detailed information about participating towns, schools, and police departments. Using this technology to collect information saves time and staff resources. As shown in Table 1, recent developments and advances in a variety of computer software programs can also increase the speed and accuracy of completing large labor-intensive tasks. Technology that enables researchers to digitally archive data can help to solve immediate storage problems and can also preserve data for long periods of time in a readily accessible format. Network computer technology allows for efficient processing and sharing of information within the research team, as well as with participating communities. Utilizing these technologies helped our research team process data quickly and report information back to the communities in an efficient and effective manner. These technologies permit our small research team to conduct a large-scale, multi-community tobacco prevention project.

Despite the obvious advantages offered by technology, there are some limitations. While the Internet provides a wealth of information, some of this information can be unreliable or dated. Sophisticated software applications required our project to invest resources to set up, to train staff, and to maintain the technology. Consequently, the resources

TABLE 1. Computer Software to Facilitate Community Research

Name	Publisher	Description
BusinessMAP III	Environmental Systems Research Institute	Computer-aided mapping program that permits the user to represent various types of information geographically.
TELEform	Cardiff Software Inc.	Information capture system that permits the user to design data collection forms, scan the data into the computer, verify inaccurate responses, and export the data to a statistical software program.
Access	Microsoft	Relational database program that permits the user to combine information contained in multiple spreadsheets into one system.
Biblioscape	CG Information	Specialized reference management software that permits the user to categorize, search, and manage large amounts of reference material.

invested in the technology must be less than the resources saved in order for the technology to be efficient. Heavy reliance on complicated technologies also puts the project at risk for a sudden work stoppage when a software application or the computer network crashes. Such instances can be very frustrating and humbling.

FUTURE DIRECTIONS

There are clear advantages and limitations to utilizing technology for community research. So far, technology has allowed our research team to complete a range of complex tasks more efficiently, which provides more resources for project implementation. While this paper does not exhaust the full range of applications of technology in community research, it demonstrates many opportunities for researchers to take advantage of existing technology to improve the research process. Our research team constantly looks for new developments in technology that we can apply to our work to improve our research and increase our efficiency. For example, we are considering using the Internet to collect the student survey data because of the amount of time and resources it would save our research team. This procedure would have students use the computer lab at their school to log onto a secure Web site and complete the survey. Unfortunately, there is no published research on the reliability and validity of collecting tobacco, alcohol, and other drug use information from youth over the Internet. Finally, our research team is working to enhance our operation further by eliminating some of the problems we currently experience because of the technological limitations noted earlier.

REFERENCES

American Psychological Association. (1993). Record keeping guidelines. *American Psychologist, 48*(9), 984-986.

Bracht, N., & Kingsbury, L. (1990). Community organization principles in health promotion. *Health Promotion at the Community Level*, 66-86.

Cardiff Software Inc. (1991). TELEform Elite (Version 7) [Computer software]. Vista, CA: Cardiff Software Inc.

CG Information. (1997). Biblioscape (Version 4) [Computer software]. Alpharetta, GA: CG Information.

Cohen, L. (2001). Click on the dotted line: 'E-signatures' come of age and make the future of e-commerce a little brighter. *New Jersey Law Journal, 80*(2), 101-105.

Curie, C. J., Pokorny, S. B., Jason, L. A., Schoeny, M. E., & Townsend, S. M. (2002). An examination of factors influencing illegal tobacco sales to minors. *Journal of Prevention & Intervention in the Community, 24*, 63-76.

Engstrom, M., Jason, L. A., Townsend, S. M., Pokorny, S. B., & Curie, C. J. (2002). Community readiness for prevention: Applying stage theory to multi-community interventions. *Journal of Prevention & Intervention in the Community, 24*, 29-46.

Environmental Systems Research Institute. (1996). *BusinessMAP PRO* (Version 2.0) [Computer software]. Richardson, TX: Environmental Systems Research Institute.

Environmental Systems Research Institute. (2002). *BusinessMAP 3* [Computer software]. Richardson, TX: Environmental Systems Research Institute.

Goldsborough, R. (2001). Staking your claim on the Web. *Community College Week, 13*, 13.

Illinois State Board of Education. (2001). *Illinois School Report Card* [Data file]. Available from Illinois State Board of Education Web site, *http://www.isbe.state.il.us*

Jason, L. A., & Pokorny, S. B. (Eds.). (2002). *Preventing youth access to tobacco*. New York: Haworth.

Jason, L. A., Pokorny, S. B., & Schoeny, M. (2003). Evaluating the effects of enforcements and fines on youth smoking. *Critical Public Health, 13*, 33-45.

Ji, P. Y., Pokorny, S. B., Blaszkowski, E., Jason, L. A., & Rabin-Belyaev, O. (2002). Examining risks for minors participating in tobacco purchase attempts. *Journal of Prevention & Intervention in the Community, 24*, 77-85.

Jorgensen, C. K., & Karlsmose, B. (1998). Validation of automated forms processing: A comparison of Teleform™ with manual data entry. *Computers in Biology and Medicine, 28*(6), 659-667.

Lindsay, W. (2000). The Internet: An aid to student research or a source of frustration? *Journal of Educational Media, 25*, 115-129.

Nazarali-Stranieri, F. (2000). The geography of technological progress. *Change Exchange, 2*, 3-5.

Perry, R. (2000). Small cities can meet e-service challenges. *American City & County, 115*, 10.

Pokorny, S. B., Townsend, S. M., Jason, L.A., Lautenschlager, H., & Smith, R. (2002). Measuring the quality of laws limiting youth access to tobacco. *Journal of Prevention & Intervention in the Community, 24*, 15-27.

Samuel, J. (2000). Medium in search of a message. *Change Exchange, 2*, 16-18.

Strover, S. (2001). Rural Internet connectivity. *Telecommunications Policy, 25*, 331-348.

Townsend, S. M., Pokorny, S. B., Jason, L. A., Curie, C. J., & Schoeny, M. E. (2002). An assessment of the relationship between the quality of school-based tobacco prevention programs and youth tobacco use. *Journal of Prevention & Intervention in the Community, 24*, 47-61.

U.S. Census Bureau. (2000). American Fact Finder [Data file]. Available from U.S. Census Bureau Web site, *http://factfinder.census.gov/servlet/BasicFactsServlet*

Wittie, R. A., & Winn, J. K. (2000). Electronic records and signatures under the federal E-Sign legislation and the UETA. *The Business Lawyer, 56*, 293-351.

Community Building with Technology: The Development of Collaborative Community Technology Initiatives in a Mid-Size City

Courtney C. Shull
Bill Berkowitz

University of Massachusetts Lowell

SUMMARY. This article describes the creation and development of community technology initiatives in Lowell, Massachusetts, a historically poor and ethnically diverse mid-size city. In the past two years, many organizations have joined in community-wide efforts to share information and resources electronically and to launch new electronic technology projects. Recent initiatives include a comprehensive computerized public database of area-wide health and human service programs, a centralized multi-purpose community Web site, and a new inter-agency community technology collaborative. This article reviews

---

Address correspondence to: Bill Berkowitz, Department of Psychology, University of Massachusetts Lowell South Campus, One University Avenue, Lowell, MA 01854 (E-mail: Bill_Berkowitz@uml.edu).

The authors wish to extend special thanks to Jane Benfey of the Greater Lowell Family Resource Collaborative for her comments on a previous draft of this article, and to Ms. Benfey and Felicia Sullivan of the Lowell Telecommunications Corporation for their ongoing guidance and support of the initiatives described here.

[Haworth co-indexing entry note]: "Community Building with Technology: The Development of Collaborative Community Technology Initiatives in a Mid-Size City." Shull, Courtney C., and Bill Berkowitz. Co-published simultaneously in *Journal of Prevention & Intervention in the Community* (The Haworth Press, Inc.) Vol. 29, No. 1/2, 2005, pp. 29-41; and: *Technology Applications in Prevention* (ed: Steven Godin) The Haworth Press, Inc., 2005, pp. 29-41. Single or multiple copies of this article are available for a fee from The Haworth Document Delivery Service [1-800-HAWORTH, 9:00 a.m. - 5:00 p.m. (EST). E-mail address: docdelivery@haworthpress.com].

Digital Object Identifier: 10.1300/J005v29n01_03

these activities and describes general lessons learned in electronic community building that may apply to other communities. *[Article copies available for a fee from The Haworth Document Delivery Service: 1-800-HAWORTH. E-mail address: <docdelivery@haworthpress.com> Website: <http://www. HaworthPress.com> © 2005 by The Haworth Press, Inc. All rights reserved.]*

KEYWORDS. Internet, capacity-building, Community Tool Box, technology

Community agencies and organizations have traditionally worked separately to provide resources and services for their residents. In recent years, however, providers have become more interested in coordinating services so as to increase efficiency and avoid duplication. To achieve such goals, local collaboratives have frequently been developed. Often, these collaboratives are based on specific issues; for example, many communities will have coalitions focusing on parenting, substance abuse, youth, housing, or other local interests.

With recent fiscal cutbacks and service reductions affecting many communities, and providers within those communities, it has become essential to find innovative ways to utilize and share resources. One such way is to apply the collaborative model to electronic technology. The original mission of this project was to identify and develop electronic technology resources to prevent social problems and create a healthier community. One still-undeveloped resource in our community, and probably in many other communities, is the Internet.

Most people know that they can use the Internet to send and receive e-mail, chat with friends, and do shopping, but many do not realize that the same Internet can become a repository for a whole host of community-building tools. As a basic example, local organizations can create Web sites to advertise programs. However, the potential of community building on the Web goes far beyond basic marketing. Community builders can take the infinite information potential found on the Web and create a new type of supportive community: a virtual community (Rheingold, 1993). Information technology can create such a community not by gathering people at a common geographic location, but through their participation in computer networks (London, 1997). These networks can strengthen community bonds. They collate not only masses of information, but also masses of people to use them. Their possibilities are limitless.

A community technology collaborative in particular can use the Internet to enhance everyone's networking experience (Dezendorf & Green, 2000). For instance, members of a local collaborative may gather bi-monthly to interact with colleagues working for similar goals. However, people do not come simply to interact; they want to exchange information, explore possibilities of reciprocity, and work within a given economy (London, 1997). With these points in mind, the present project explores how electronic technology can be used to maximize the value of service time and resources.

A community technology collaborative can and should be based upon many of the central premises of community psychology. To begin with, the success of the initiative will depend upon people's ability first to form and then to identify with the collaborative's mission or goal. Beyond that, the collaborative should be open to everyone; reflect the local culture; respond to stated needs; stimulate participation; bring together members of the community; and promote debate to resolve shared issues (cf. Kim, 2000). Next, the initiative's leaders and members should identify the competencies and strengths in their collaborative's network, while at the same time looking beyond the existing network for additional solutions (Morino, 1994). In simpler terms, those leaders and members should know their community's assets and work with them, but continue to think outside the box.

Accordingly, the goals of the present project were to identify electronic technology activities in our community, to strengthen them, and to develop new collaborative efforts. The text below begins with a description of the our home community and its prior technological status; it then records methods used to collect information, describes resulting initiatives taken to expand technological capacity, and notes some of their outcomes. Several challenges faced and lessons learned about developing Internet-based community-building initiatives are then highlighted, which may be applicable to other communities wishing to develop initiatives of their own.

PROCEDURE

The Community Setting

This community-building project took place in Lowell, Massachusetts. Lowell is a middle-sized city, with a population of about 100,000, located 30 miles northwest of Boston; historically, it is a former mill city as well as a traditional city for immigrants. Despite some economic and cultural revival in recent years, Lowell is still regarded as one of the most economically disadvantaged cities in the state. Lowell may also be the most ethnically diverse community of its size in America; it has the largest Cambodian population (25,000-30,000) in the United States, together with significant populations of Latinos and people of Portuguese background (about 15,000 each), complemented by the new arrival of about 5,000 people of African descent.

Prior Technological Status

Prior to the start of this project, few successful inter-agency attempts to utilize electronic technology had occurred. There were, however, at least three interested local organizations, similar to those that might be present in other communities, and whose existence provided an impetus for development:

1. the University of Massachusetts Lowell, with both an historically strong School of Engineering and a graduate program in Community Psychology committed to community outreach and community building;
2. the Lowell Telecommunications Corporation, a downtown media and technology center with public computer facilities and video and cable television production capabilities, committed to community development through electronic technology education and training;
3. the Nonprofit Alliance of Greater Lowell, a loose organization of community service agencies in the city, with specific interests in collaboration and coordination.

Despite the presence of these organizations and the resources they could provide, electronic technology development was limited in large part because of the lack of centralized coordinating structures. This investigation was therefore undertaken to more current conditions more formally, to determine needs, and to identify collaborative activities and structures best designed to meet those needs.

Methods of Investigation

Field Observations. The first phase of data collection was through simple field observation of three community-based meetings. Each meeting, with different institutional sponsorship, gathered community leaders and service providers to discuss community issues currently being faced. Common themes voiced by representatives at all meetings were the needs for expanded Internet awareness, education, and training, and the parallel need for better technology-based tools.

Surveys. A second investigation phase involved collection of survey data from a broader range of community-based organizations. The Nonprofit Alliance of Greater Lowell distributed these surveys to more than 30 local agency leaders. Results confirmed those of the earlier meetings. They also pointed to gaps in knowledge about other local programs and revealed increasing amounts of program duplication.

Data Collection on Existing Initiatives. Finally, the first investigator facilitated a follow-up meeting to collect data on other local Web-based community initiatives. The meeting was held at a local restaurant to provide an informal atmosphere. The diverse representatives at this meeting, gathered together for the first time, included staff from local technology organizations, service groups, local libraries, community health centers, the university, and cultural groups. After collection of information, there was discussion about barriers to providing community-wide technology services and brainstorming about how to overcome those barriers. The results of this meeting created the foundation for the beginning of more collaborative efforts, as noted below.

RESULTS

Based upon these assessments, and emerging from these meetings, a number of new collaborative initiatives using electronic technology were undertaken during the past two years. We describe three of the most significant in this section.

The Merrimack Valley Hub

The Merrimack Valley Hub is a public online data bank of local nonprofit services and resources. The site was developed both to offer service providers an accurate database for making referrals, and also to empower community members by supplying free and easy access to information about resources ranging from foster care and education opportunities to support groups and housing information. The Hub, which is based upon "IRis for the Web" software, was launched in December 2001 through a collaboration of The Greater Lowell Family Resource

Collaborative, Lowell Weed and Seed (an anti-crime organization), New Beginnings (a local agency providing computer and job training skills), and the University of Massachusetts Lowell, but also with the active support of many other local agencies, groups, and individuals.

The heart of the Hub is a Web site, located at www.MVHub.com, that enables users to access information about community-based and regional programs using a variety of different search methods. Once connected to the site, a user can search for resources either drawing upon over 300 preselected visible service categories, or upon self-generated keywords. The site may also be searched alphabetically, by program name, by sponsoring agency, by city name, or by zip code. All resource listings generated through any of the above searches contain information on program eligibility, areas served, hours of operation, costs, waiting lists (if any), languages spoken, public transportation, handicapped accessibility, volunteer opportunities, other requirements or conditions of service, and detailed contact information, including e-mail addresses. Maps showing the precise site location can be downloaded; English-to-Spanish translation is also available.

The Hub site, which is updated regularly, is set up to provide the easiest access possible for a user to find out what programs are available to serve his or her own needs. Information about more than 200 local health and human service programs is posted. The site is the first known project of its kind in the state; it is unique because it provides comprehensive and free information about services available in the Merrimack Valley to anyone with an Internet connection.

A Better Lowell

A Better Lowell, another Web site located at www.AbetterLowell.org, complements the Merrimack Valley Hub (to which it is linked) by providing a broad variety of more interactive tools. The first investigator created this site on the basis of the needs assessments previously described. Service providers in general had reported not knowing what programs were going on in other agencies, and feared duplication of programs and services. They expressed interest in communicating more regularly with other community leaders, but time constraints made it difficult for this type of interaction to occur.

Throughout the development and pilot test phases of A Better Lowell, potential users offered helpful feedback for tools and formats to include. Many expressed interest not only in making site submissions but also offered suggestions on how to make it better. As a result, the A

Better Lowell site was launched in early 2002, with joint sponsorship from the University of Massachusetts Lowell, which has provided staff resources to facilitate site development, and from the Lowell Telecommunications Corporation, which has supplied training and technical assistance in site implementation. The site contains the following key features.

Home Page. Besides supplying a basic navigational framework, the home page also contains a periodically rotating feature spotlighting the accomplishments of local programs. In addition, it affords contact and tracking information for users to continue reviewing and making suggestions for the site.

Community Tools Page. The community tools page provides a changing series of community-building resources and instruction. As an example, one of the first tools featured was on creative program development; the page described key factors in such development and the related how-to's. For more detailed information on the featured tool as well as overheads for teaching, a link to the Community Tool Box was created. The Community Tool Box, based at the University of Kansas and located at ctb.ku.edu, is a national community-building Internet initiative that provides more than 250 modular sections on different community health and development topics (cf. Schultz et al., 2000).

Jobs and Volunteer Opportunities Page. This page was created to view and share job and volunteer opportunities around the community. Postings are listed and categorized by the submitting agency or organization. The submission and application processes are simplified by a contact link provided right on the page.

Calendar Page. The community calendar page provides agencies a space to post programs, trainings, and events in one centralized location–a major benefit in coordinating community events. The format of the page has invisible tag links to make viewing simpler. Calendar submissions are made directly on the screen in identical fashion as the job and volunteer page.

"Ask an Advisor" Page. This page was added in order to provide users with a place to get personalized information and support related to particular community-building questions they might have. Users are invited to click on the contact link and submit their questions to a local community development specialist; the specialist then delivers a customized response to the submitter. The model here follows one previously used with success by NetWellness, at www.netwellness.org, a well-known health information site.

Community Message Board Page. To use this feature, the user simply clicks on a message board icon. The boards are used for interaction between agencies and community members. Someone might need suggestions about an upcoming program, for instance, or want feedback on a recent community event. The user could submit his or her query and have other community site users respond in public forum. The page can also be used to post community meeting notes for curious community members to read and find out about current organizational activities.

"First Monday." AbetterLowell.org also produced an e-mailed based community newsletter ("First Monday"). This newsletter is unique because it not only spotlights key events and gives organizational profiles, but also includes community perspectives. The newsletter collected voices from the community to comment on Lowell, and offer their vision for Lowell's future. First Monday was distributed via e-mail to a list of about 225 local service providers. Reader feedback was very positive: one community leader noted, "First Monday provides a unique perspective about what it is like to live in Lowell, while giving an outlet to providers and residents to share their ideas and visions."

Technology Action Group

As a direct result of the commitments of those involved with the programs above, a new community-wide Technology Action Group (TAG) was formed. Prior to TAG, community technology leaders communicated with each other informally; one might send a simple e-mail to another to provide updates on project progress. This was a useful beginning arrangement, but it did not prevent duplication of ideas, share resources, or help in overall community problem solving.

TAG was formally established in February 2003 with a core group of ten members, including community technology professionals, library administrators, university staff, city management officials, local health and human service managers, and representatives of ethnic and cultural coalitions. While each member represents a different sector of the community, all have interest in moving community technology forward. The stated mission of the group, adopted early in 2003, is "to enhance the use of information technology in the community by sharing resources, identifying needs, and reducing program duplication."

TAG has already addressed some barriers to providing community technology services and sharing information both within the group and within the community. Currently the group is helping to sustain and expand current community technology projects, such as the Merrimack

Valley Hub. In coming months, the group will continue to investigate technology needs and develop new efforts on a regularly scheduled basis.

DISCUSSION

We believe the electronic technology advances in our community described above have been noteworthy. The contrast with the situation as it existed only two or three years ago is especially revealing. For example, up until that time, printed resource guides were the only comprehensive source of local community service information. Two significant problems, however, were associated with these guides. First, they became outdated very quickly, yet they could be produced only every few years because of high time and dollar costs. Second, the printed resource guides did not adequately reach their intended audience; instead, they tended to be distributed primarily to institutions, such as libraries, schools, and service providers themselves. Thus, the people who could most use the guides were the least likely to receive them.

Electronic technology has provided an effective way to address these and other concerns. Since Lowell has several programs that make computers available to the public at community sites, initiatives such as the Merrimack Valley Hub now serve lower-income or less computer-oriented populations by fostering an expanded awareness of local community services, as well as something they may never have had before–the ability to find their own services instead of relying on referrals from others. In addition, interactive efforts such as A Better Lowell stimulate both community participation as well as formal and informal linkages between residents and service providers.

Much of the purpose of this article, though, is to share not only our results but also our lessons learned with other communities–especially middle- or lower-income communities without great material resources. So we continue this discussion section by highlighting some of the main challenges we encountered and some of the key principles that we believe helped make our work successful.

Challenges

Perhaps not surprisingly, many of the challenges we faced centered less on technology as such, and more on organizational behavior and human relationships.

First, institutional inertia had to be overcome; while nonprofit leaders may see the theoretical advantages of collaborating, in daily practice it is often easier to simply attend to one's organizational business and "cultivate one's own garden."

Second, trust among these leaders needed to be established, or in some cases, reestablished. Previous attempts to create similar Internet sites and databases had failed. Leaders needed to be convinced that this effort would succeed in order for them to lend their support or offer their participation.

Third, nonprofit leaders almost always have multiple and competing demands on their time, especially in a cutback economy with increasing service needs, where there is relentless pressure to maintain services with fewer resources. Even those wanting to collaborate, and even those who had agreed to become part of a collaborative, would find it hard to agree on a simple common meeting time (for even though much of the collaborative work could be done electronically, some face-to-face meetings were still felt to be necessary).

These types of challenges are common in many collaboratives and coalitions, irrespective of content or type (e.g., Berkowitz & Wolff, 2000). They can best be overcome by high amounts of motivation and tenacity from the collaborative's leadership, combined with the skilled application of human relationship principles, as detailed below.

One additional challenge was more technical in nature, and ironically connected to electronic technology itself. When resource data for the Merrimack Valley Hub site were being collected, some agency contacts ignored our initial e-mailed requests–perhaps not due to lack of interest, but rather because of the many electronic communications they had to contend with. Some agencies required as many as ten e-mails or phone calls before responses were received. The same issue has carried over into obtaining accurate program updates; for when programs and services are being cut, responding to outside informational requests is not a priority. We learned to meet this challenge by persisting, by developing multiple contacts within each identified program, and by going to the top of the agency hierarchy when necessary.

Lessons

Many of the developmental lessons we learned (or relearned) were also organizational as well as technological in nature; again, they apply to many other forms of collaborative efforts, and can be simply stated.

First, as with other collaborative community initiatives, one needs to have a dedicated core group of people committed to implementing the group's mission. These people should ideally have a determination and a passion for building community, in this case electronically.

Second, it is essential to identify partners who might want to be involved. We were able to find them through our outreach efforts, and then to nurture their commitment. This was crucial, since even those not formally joining our collaborative still contributed useful suggestions and did not feel that their turf had been invaded. As a result, they have become active allies, rather than passive bystanders, or worse, opponents.

Third, one must continue to assess the needs of the community as reported by both service providers and residents. Our work involved a series of informal meetings, observations, and survey results, first to develop individual projects, then the Technology Action Group. Individual projects involved residents and on-site users to evaluate project effectiveness. This process helped to create a sense of ownership among participants. That is, when users saw their input incorporated into projects, they became motivated to continue their participation and contributions to project development.

Fourth, as a result of these assessments, each individual technology initiative must keep evolving. The core group also needs to keep abreast of changing technology and to create new local technology tools from ideas that are voiced by the users. A local example of this has been the creation of an all-inclusive and centralized community calendar.

Fifth, and perhaps obviously, it is most important to have community support. Community members need to feel as they are part of the projects, so that they will continue to provide input and interact with one another using the tools provided. Without the active support of the community, no electronic initiative, nor any other initiative, will be able to work at its best.

The combined application of these principles has, we believe, led to the overall success of our collaborative effort. Because many community leaders and members have been involved in providing ideas for our community initiatives, the responsibility is genuinely shared. Agencies continue to contact us to provide submissions and suggestions. Participation in the Technology Action Group and other related future efforts is expected to grow.

FUTURE DIRECTIONS

We are optimistic about the future of electronic technology collaboration in our community. Despite cutbacks and resource limits, the Technology Action Group is continuing to develop and implement a community technology vision for Lowell. Through its own efforts, and the efforts of its partner organizations, some newer initiatives not previously mentioned have begun to take hold:

- The Graduate Program in Community Psychology at the University has begun the compilation and potential distribution of a more inclusive community e-mail list, including hundreds of local organizational contacts that are not current members of the Nonprofit Alliance and not electronically connected with other groups.
- The University itself has added an "e-community" feature to its own Web site, where community organizations can freely post organizational profiles and other promotional information.
- The Community Software Lab, a new collaboration between the Lowell Telecommunications Corporation and the Computer Science Department at the University, has become involved in building and modifying software, constructing interactive forms, and designing and hosting Web sites for nonprofit community organizations. Our new community calendar format is one local example.
- The Nonprofit Alliance of Greater Lowell has added a well-trafficked listserv, an online membership directory, and an electronic magazine of its own. These additions have helped it assume a much stronger advocacy role.
- The Technology Action Group is investigating the publication of resource information on the Hub site in compact disc format for those community users who might not have easy access to the Internet.
- More generally, the Technology Action Group will be broadening its scope by surveying the needs of community groups that presently make minimal use of technology, and by seeking new ways to serve them and to incorporate their opinions and expertise.
- Finally, the Technology Action Group, with operational leadership from the Lowell Telecommunications Corporation, is working to develop a single central community Web portal, designed "to provide all the information you could want or need" about the community. It is possible that the Merrimack Valley Hub, A Better Lowell, and the Nonprofit Alliance will all become components of this unified technology source.

Through these combined technology initiatives already in place, and through others now emerging or on the horizon, we are closer to the day when Lowell–and, hopefully, communities similar to Lowell–will have universal computer access; when anyone wishing to know or learn about community resources or services can easily do so; when everyone's viewpoints and expertise can be freely shared; when new programs and initiatives will continually arise to meet resident and provider needs; when new collaborations will spring up to implement those initiatives; and when electronic community development will confer measurable and significant individual and community benefits to complement and enhance those that result from face-to-face human interaction.

REFERENCES

Berkowitz, B., & Wolff, T. (2000). *The spirit of the coalition.* Washington, D.C.: American Public Health Association.
Dezendorf, P. K., & Green, R. K. (2000). Promoting computer-mediated communications in community coalitions. *Journal of Technology in Human Services, 17* (2-3), 217-236.
Homan, M. S. (1999). *Promoting community change: Making it happen in the real world* (2nd ed.). Pacific Grove, CA: Brooks/Cole.
Kim, A. J. (2000). *Community building on the web: Secret strategies for successful online communities.* Berkeley, CA: Peachpit Press.
London, S. (1997). Civic networks: Building community on the net. [Paper prepared for Kettering Foundation; accessible at *http://www.scottlondon.com/reports/networks.html.*]
Morino, M. (1994). Assessment and evolution of community networking. [Paper presented at "The Ties that Bind" conference on building community networks.]
Rheingold, H. (1993). A slice of life in my virtual community. In Harasim, L. M. (Ed.), *Global networks: Computers and international communication* (p. 64). Cambridge: MIT Press.
Schultz, J. A., Fawcett, S. B., Francisco, V. T., Wolff, T., Berkowitz, B. R., & Nagy, G. (2000). The Community Tool Box: Using the Internet to support the work of community health and development. *Journal of Technology in Human Services, 17* (2-3), 193-215.

PROJECT-RELATED WEBSITES

A Better Lowell	*http://www.abetterlowell.org*
Community Tool Box	*http://ctb.ku.edu*
Lowell Telecommunications Corporation	*http://www.ltc.org*
Merrimack Valley Hub	*http://www.MVHub.com*
NetWellness	*http://www.netwellness.org*
Nonprofit Alliance of Greater Lowell	*http://www.npagl.org*
Technology Action Group	*http://www.tag.ltc.org*
University of Massachusetts Lowell	*http://www.uml.edu*

(For additional background information on other community technology projects, see also various issues of the *Community Technology Review*, online at *www.comtechreview.org*)

Applying Web-Based
Survey Design Standards

Scott Crawford

MSIResearch

Sean Esteban McCabe

University of Michigan

Duston Pope

MSIResearch

SUMMARY. Web-based surveys are used as research tools in a wide range of disciplines. Web-based surveys present a unique set of challenges concerning survey design, not known in previous survey modes. The flexibility of screen design allows for Web-based surveys to take on many appearances, some having a negative impact on data quality. In this article, we propose and illustrate several Web-based survey design standards developed by researchers based on several projects involving Web-based surveys. These standards have been developed from theory and practice and should provide practical advice for researchers and a platform for future research in Web-based survey design. *[Article copies available for a fee from The Haworth Document Delivery Service: 1-800-HAWORTH. E-mail address:*

Address correspondence to: Scott Crawford, Survey Sciences Group, LLC, 2232 South Main Street #473, Ann Arbor, MI 48103-6938.

[Haworth co-indexing entry note]: "Applying Web-Based Survey Design Standards." Crawford, Scott, Sean Esteban McCabe, and Duston Pope. Co-published simultaneously in *Journal of Prevention & Intervention in the Community* (The Haworth Press, Inc.) Vol. 29, No. 1/2, 2005, pp. 43-66; and: *Technology Applications in Prevention* (ed: Steven Godin) The Haworth Press, Inc., 2005, pp. 43-66. Single or multiple copies of this article are available for a fee from The Haworth Document Delivery Service [1-800-HAWORTH, 9:00 a.m. - 5:00 p.m. (EST). E-mail address: docdelivery@haworthpress.com].

http://www.haworthpress.com/web/JPIC
Digital Object Identifier: 10.1300/J005v29n01_04

KEYWORDS. Internet, Web-based surveys, evaluation, human factors, Web-standards

INTRODUCTION

The day has arrived where social scientists and evaluation researchers can use the Internet as an effective tool in their work. Researchers are now using Web-based surveys in support of their needs assessments and evaluation research efforts. The debate has shifted from whether or not the Internet has a place in survey research to how the technology can be best utilized to maximize quality (Couper, 2000; Vehovar et al. 2001), and improve efficiency or reduce costs (Crawford et al., 2002). In this article, we will look closely at design issues in Web-based surveys for collecting social science data. In the past, various data collection strategies were explored and their error structures became understood over time (Groves et al., 1988). Web-based surveys are now going through similar study. In this article we will describe what goes into good quality Web-based survey design.

As researchers use the Web as a venue for data collection, they must develop a new set of standards for the construction of computer-assisted surveys. With interviewer-administered computer-assisted surveys, little attention has been given to the design of the survey instrument. Weaknesses in the designs of computer-assisted surveys were frequently dealt with by providing training to interviewers to compensate for the problem. Given a variety of software limitations and other influences, survey research organizations made adjustments by developing a culture that promoted a mantra of "We can just train the interviewers around this problem." However, with the evolution of the Internet as a survey research tool, the use of interviewers to compensate for design flaws in computer-assisted surveys fielded on the Web is not an option. Web-researchers must re-focus their attention on the development of an efficacious interface that increases internal validity of Web-based surveys.

We will make the case for researchers to develop a set of standards for the construction of Web-based surveys. The development of self-administered questionnaires and some first steps towards defining principals for Web-based surveys has been well documented and continues to be important in the evolution of Web-based surveys (Dillman, 2000).

The future, we argue, will come in a survey development focus that emphasizes the importance of the interface, the design, and the functionality of Web-based surveys.

We will close this article by providing two examples of pilot studies in which the standards discussed in this paper were implemented in intervention and prevention research. The studies demonstrate how one can apply Web-based data collections to real research problems and provide evidence that with a carefully thought through design, one can expect the same level of quality in the data collection as with traditional modes. We also note where the studies helped to improve the standards we routinely employ in Web-based surveys.

A Case for Standards

Baker et al. (2003) has taken note of the complexities involved in the testing of Web-based surveys. They have looked at Web-based survey systems as including six basic components: a respondent interface, questions and answers, logic and functionality, a respondent environment, the survey software, and the supporting hardware infrastructure. They clearly demonstrate the added complexity of Web-based surveys over traditional computer-assisted surveys. In this manuscript, we will focus our attention on reducing the complexities of the respondent interface and environment, as these two alone will drive the culture shift to focus on survey design.

The nature of the Web is that it breaks down time and space barriers. Survey researchers can reach respondents wherever they are, at whatever time is most convenient to the respondent. Unfortunately, this benefit adds to the complexity of the unknowns of varying respondents' interface and environment in which they take the survey.

Web-based surveys, by definition, are administered via the World Wide Web (WWW). They use Web browser, operating system, and hardware technologies to provide a platform on which the survey is presented to the respondent. Because of the variability involved, however, it is not realistic to expect everyone to have equally comparable environments from which to take a Web-based survey. Further, even if respondents do have identical systems, the nature of the technology allows for a customization of preferences, compounding the problem for those interested in maintaining consistency in survey administration.

Although complex, all variations in software and preference settings can be known and thoroughly evaluated to determine their impact on the respondents' experience. In an ideal world with unlimited resources, an evaluation would take place using all possible combinations, prior to launching any Web-based survey. A more realistic approach includes a full evaluation of each component of a Web-based survey that is commonly utilized. Take as an example a single response option question. Such a question design could be created, standardized, and then thoroughly tested. So long as the change to the tested design remains with question or response content and not in its layout or interface, it would be safe to assume that this question will present as desired on the great variety of user configurations that exist.

With standards, identifying new quality issues becomes easier, as patterns may emerge where designs impact data quality. For example, if it is noted that a high rate of respondent "break-offs" (where respondents leave a survey unfinished) take place at a specific question type, standards allow the researcher to quickly identify possible causes by narrowing the scope of possibilities to the technologies involved in the standard application of the question.

Standards can also increase the efficiency of Web-based surveys. Programmers can build templates, libraries, and automated systems that take questionnaire specifications and turn them into the basis of a Web-based survey.

Most importantly, standards help promote consistency and quality in Web-based surveys to facilitate comparisons across studies. Standards for Web-based survey design can be viewed in a similar way as the structure around a structured interview. With established standards, we know that a question is not only worded the same way for each respondent, but it is also presented (or asked) similarly for every respondent.

The process of developing standards for Web-based survey design closely follows most models of scientific exploration. Beginning with theories of how to best collect survey data using the Web, researchers must find the best application of such theories taking into consideration their available resources. As designs are implemented, they are tested empirically. Such tests will either confirm the existing standard, or suggest new standards are required. Under this process, standards will continually grow and improve. It is *not* desirable for a set of standards to be imposed on the field of survey research to be adopted blindly as *the way* to conduct Web-based surveys. It is clear that the survey data collection process is becoming more and more customized, focusing on individual needs of the respondent and researcher. Standards should always be created with such flexibility in mind.

Web-based survey standards fall into four categories: screen design, questionnaire writing, respondent communications, and process standards. Screen design standards are arguably where the most deviation from known data collection methodologies exists, and thus will serve as the focus of this article. The following screen design standards have been developed over the past seven years of conducting Web-based surveys. We would like to emphasize that these standards are specific to our organization, to the resources it maintains, and influenced by the typical respondent that is included in surveys we conduct.

In the presentation of these standards, we will note where clear empirical evidence pointing at issues with data quality has been used to establish the existing standard. However, many of the standards have yet to be fully tested in empirical experiments across a broad range of sub-populations. Until such time as they are tested, we can only rely upon our opinion in how we have applied theoretical knowledge to the practice of Web-based survey research. We hope sharing these standards may be useful, but also may inspire others to dispute or support them in their own research.

Screen Design Standards

Screen design standards include guidance on the visual display of questions, responses, and supporting survey materials to the respondent. In developing standards for screen design, we have found that it is important to pay attention to self-administered survey design and implementation (Dillman, 2000), human-computer interaction (Couper, 2002), and Web site usability (Nielsen, 2000) literatures. Researchers must always consider the goals of survey research when applying knowledge gained from other fields of study, such as Web site usability. Web site usability researchers may have as an ultimate goal the attraction of people to a Web site. While such attraction is desirable in Web-based surveys, the primary goal of a Web-based survey is to get a respondent to answer all the appropriate questions as accurately as possible. So, the focus may shift from attracting attention to the site, to making the survey taking process as streamlined and easy to complete as possible with minimal distractions. Researchers should keep such differences in mind when applying literature from other fields of study to Web-based survey research.

We break screen design standards down into five sub-categories: general screen design, text, question presentation, respondent input/response format, and survey navigation/interaction. The following pages will present our standards within each sub-category.

General Screen Design

General screen design encompasses the general look and feel of the screen presentation itself. Surveys should be designed, as shown in Figure 1, to contain no background color or images. Background colors may create a problem with contrast where text may become difficult to read. Background images may also increase download time, which, in turn, can be problematic with respondents who have dial-up Internet connections.

When used, a graphic or logo may be presented using a small (in screen space size and file size) graphic located in the upper left corner of the screen. The purpose of such a graphic should be limited to maintaining a desired look and feel of the survey instrument in connection with the data collection organization or sponsor of the research. Care must be taken to using graphics that will not influence how respondents respond to the survey questions. For example, if a survey were in support of an evaluation of a program geared to connect police officers with children in the community, it would *not* be a good design to include a logo that showed a friendly-looking police officer smiling at the respondent throughout the survey. The potential for the image to bias the immediate mood of the respondent, and ultimately their responses, is too great.

FIGURE 1. General Screen Design

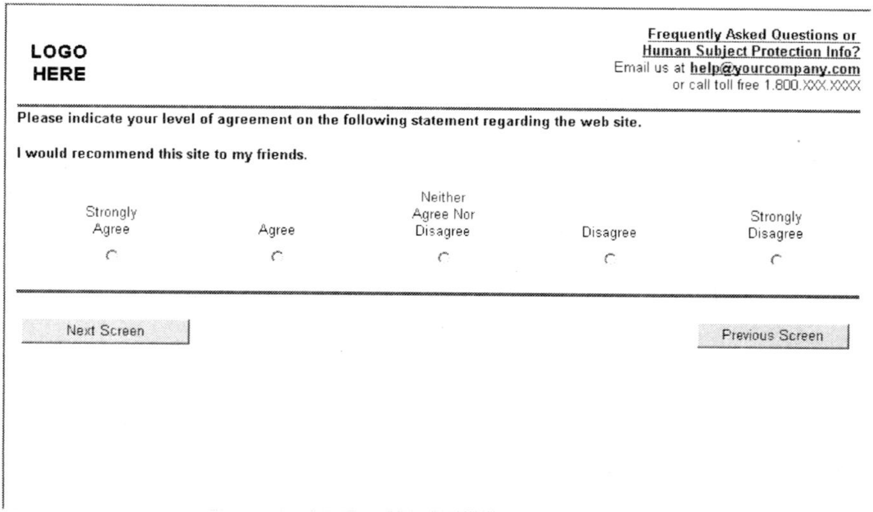

LOGO HERE

<u>Frequently Asked Questions or Human Subject Protection Info?</u>
Email us at <u>help@yourcompany.com</u>
or call toll free 1.800.XXX.XXXX

Please indicate your level of agreement on the following statement regarding the web site.

I would recommend this site to my friends.

Strongly Agree	Agree	Neither Agree Nor Disagree	Disagree	Strongly Disagree
⌀	⌀	⌀	⌀	⌀

Next Screen   Previous Screen

Also related to the standard of using a small graphic or logo, it should be noted that generally most multimedia (graphics, video, audio, or other graphical or interactive files) should not be used in Web-based surveys unless they are very small in size to allow for quick downloads on slow connections. While the proportion of Internet users connected with high speed connections (DSL, cable, T1, etc.) are increasing, as of early 2002 according to the Pew Internet & American Life Project, only 21 percent of those connected to the Internet were connected through a high speed connection.

The upper right corner of each screen should contain contact information and other supplemental information for respondents to use if they come across a problem or have a question during data collection. Frequently we place privacy or other Institutional Review Board information as a clickable link in this area. This location is always visible on every screen and will not drop off the bottom where respondents must scroll to find.

Both the logo and contact info should be placed at the top of the screen and made visible to respondents on every screen. Because the top of every screen looks the same, respondents will tend to ignore this area after a first review and focus on the content that changes. This phenomenon has been coined "Banner-Blindness" when applied to advertising banners on Web sites (Benway, 1998). In this case, what works against online marketers works for Web-based survey researchers.

The task of finding the question on each screen should be made as easy as possible for the respondents. To help identify where the logo and contact information ends, and the survey question begins, we place a thin line of separation immediately below the logo that extends the entire width of the screen. Respondents will get accustomed to knowing that they should focus their attention to the text immediately below this line to read the question. Similarly, a blue line is used to separate the questions and responses from the survey navigation buttons.

We have found that using a progress indicator (a graphic or text label that tells the respondent information about how far they have progressed though the survey) may increase respondent break-off (Crawford et al., 2000) in some situations, while others have found no such effect. (Couper et al., 2001). We hypothesize that the respondents' perception of how burdensome it will be to complete the survey has a direct correlation with how likely it will be that the respondent continues in the survey at any given moment. When respondents see a progress indicator, we believe they extrapolate the time they have taken thus far in the survey and decide on how long the survey will take overall. In a survey that begins with burdensome questions that may take longer to answer than average, such an interpretation may result in an evaluation of burden that is too high. These hypotheses have been recently supported by Conrad et al. (2003) in a study where the progress indicator was manipulated experimentally to simulate a slowing down progress indicator (where respondents received "good news" about the survey progress early in the survey), a constant progress indicator that showed a linear relationship between number of items completed and the total completion of the survey, and a speeding up progress indicator (where respondents received "bad news first"). The speeding up progress indicator created the highest break-off rate, while the slowing down indicator created the lowest. We recommend that *no progress indicators* should be used in Web-based surveys until it is better understood how to effectively use them to improve, and not hurt, completion rates.

Text

A good standard for Web-based surveys is to use black color text in a sans serif font (Arial is a common sans serif font that we prefer to use). The font size should be between 10 and 12 points, with some attention to who the population of study is in deciding on a final font size. For example, it would be important to use the larger font size of 12 points with populations that include the elderly and the visually impaired.

Use a bold font format for all questions, with response categories in regular font format. This provides the respondent with the ease of quickly identifying which portion of the written text is the question and which is the response list.

When emphasis is used, we prefer to keep it short and make it bold blue in color, as demonstrated in Figure 2. This use of color helps identify the word as important. We also recommend the use of the color red to identify error messages. Error messages should always be placed on the screen in a location where they are likely to be seen and appropriately attributed to the correct question, if there are multiple questions presented on the screen. (For an example of such a question, see Figure 5.)

While cultural norms help us in identifying red as the correct color to use in error messages, the selection of bold blue for emphasis has been a difficult one. Bold is already used as the standard format for question text, so it is not available as emphasis. Underlining text is commonly thought of as associated with hyperlinks on the Web, and thus we have

FIGURE 2. Use of Selective Emphasis and Instructions Text

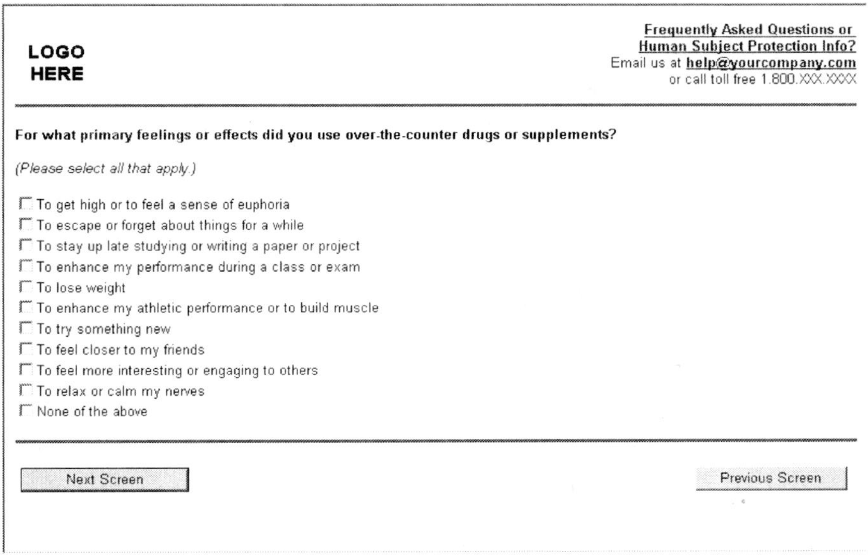
LOGO
HERE

Frequently Asked Questions or
Human Subject Protection Info?
Email us at help@yourcompany.com
or call toll free 1.800.XXX.XXXX

For what primary feelings or effects did you use over-the-counter drugs or supplements?

(Please select all that apply.)

- To get high or to feel a sense of euphoria
- To escape or forget about things for a while
- To stay up late studying or writing a paper or project
- To enhance my performance during a class or exam
- To lose weight
- To enhance my athletic performance or to build muscle
- To try something new
- To feel closer to my friends
- To feel more interesting or engaging to others
- To relax or calm my nerves
- None of the above

Next Screen

Previous Screen

avoided its use. Use of text in ALL CAPS has also been considered and is avoided primarily because it may be more difficult to read if used too frequently within a question. While we have settled on bold blue for consistency, at this point, we have found no evidence to show that there is any difference in data quality when bold blue, ALL CAPS, or underlining is used. We encourage researchers to develop means for studying and evaluating this standard, as well as the use of emphasis in general.

Instructions, meant to assist respondents in how to respond to the current question, are placed below the question text and above the response categories. They are placed in parenthesis and in an italics font format (Figure 2). This format for instructions does not draw the focus of the respondent away from the question, but still provides the necessary instruction if and when the respondent needs information about how to answer a specific question.

Question Presentation

Question presentation standards guide researchers in the overall design of how questions are presented to respondents in Web-based surveys. Unfortunately, question presentation is one of the most limiting capabilities given most survey software packages available. There is always a trade-off with resource/software availability and capability when working with highly customized systems such as those that allow researchers to field Web-based surveys.

At the core of these standards lie the distinction between an interactive and a static Web-based survey. Interactive Web-based surveys allow the researcher the flexibility of including skip logic, data validations, and other customized components to a Web-based survey that is transparent to the respondent. Static Web-based surveys follow more closely to the design and layout of paper-based surveys, with all content on one or a few scrolling screens, allowing for minimal programmatic interaction with the respondent. The operational reality of conducting Web-based surveys is that most fall somewhere in between those two extremes. The degree to which they do usually depends on the software in use and the knowledge of the programmers to stretch the capabilities of the software.

A standard we recommend for Web-based surveys, when the capability exists, is to provide only so many questions on one screen as fit without requiring the respondent to scroll down to see the navigation button(s). When required by the survey design for other reasons, we do sometimes create pages with questions that require vertical scrolling. However, *avoid designing a survey that requires horizontal scrolling* where content is off the left or right side of the visible browser window.

In an interactive Web-based survey, question numbers do not serve the same purpose as they do with assisting respondent navigation in paper-based surveys. We recommend leaving numbers off. This avoids confusion when respondents notice skip logic has skipped them past some question numbers. It also minimizes the likelihood that respondents may misinterpret the length of the survey as they have shown to do in some situations with progress indicators.

Fully labeled scale questions should be displayed vertically (Figure 3). One exception to this standard is when responses are placed in questions formatted as a grid (with column headers as the response options, and column rows presenting each unique question or evaluation statement). If the scale is not fully labeled, it should be presented horizontally below the question (Figure 4).

When grid questions are used (Figure 5), they should not exceed a total of more than 12 columns in width. All grid columns containing response options should be consistently spaced such that none stand out from others. Basic HTML presents columns to be as wide as the widest content of any cell within the column, presenting an uneven display of response op-

FIGURE 3. Vertical Scale Question Layout

**LOGO
HERE**

Frequently Asked Questions or
Human Subject Protection Info?
Email us at help@yourcompany.com
or call toll free 1.800.XXX.XXXX

What is the highest level of education completed by your mother or female guardian?

○ Less than high school
○ Completed high school
○ Some college
○ Completed college
○ Graduate or professional school
○ Does not apply
○ Rather not say

[Next Screen]   [Previous Screen]

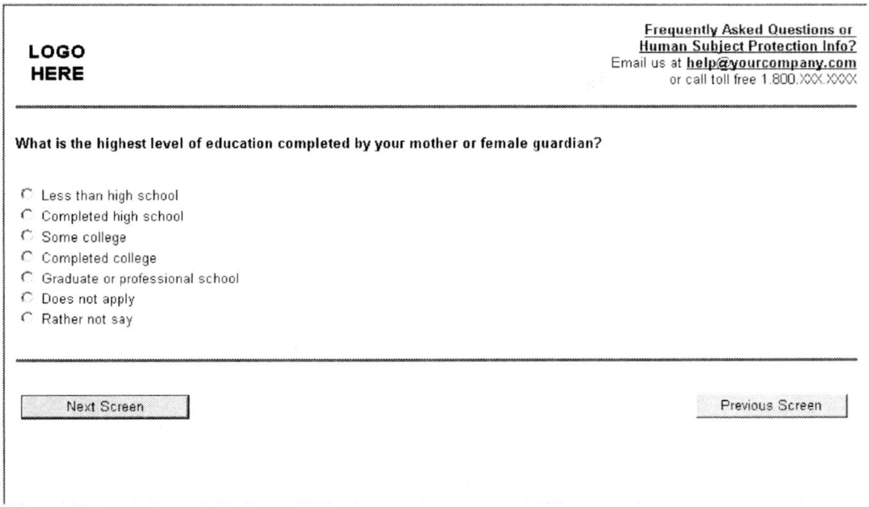

FIGURE 4. Horizontal Scale Question Layout

**LOGO
HERE**

Frequently Asked Questions or
Human Subject Protection Info?
Email us at help@yourcompany.com
or call toll free 1.800.XXX.XXXX

Overall Satisfaction

Overall, how satisfied are you with the survey?

Not Satisfied 0	1	2	3	4	5	6	7	8	9	Very Satisfied 10	N/A
○	○	○	○	○	○	○	○	○	○	○	○

[Next Screen]   [Previous Screen]

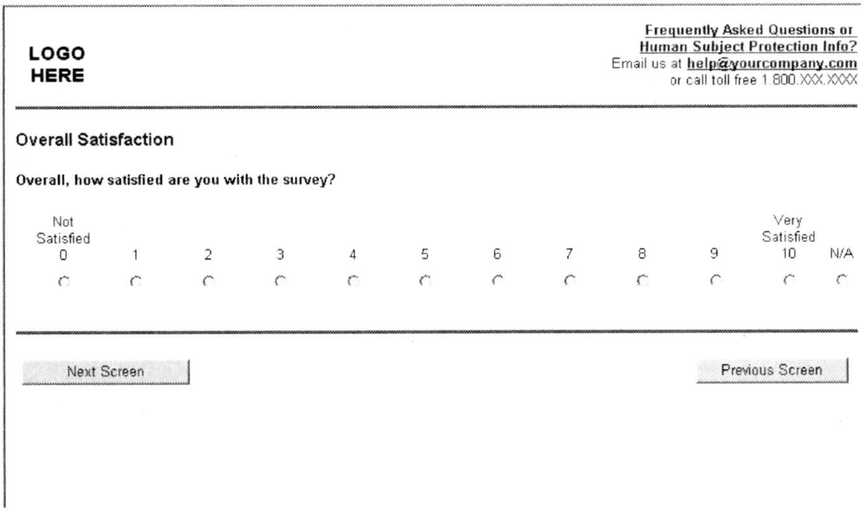

FIGURE 5. Grid Question Standards

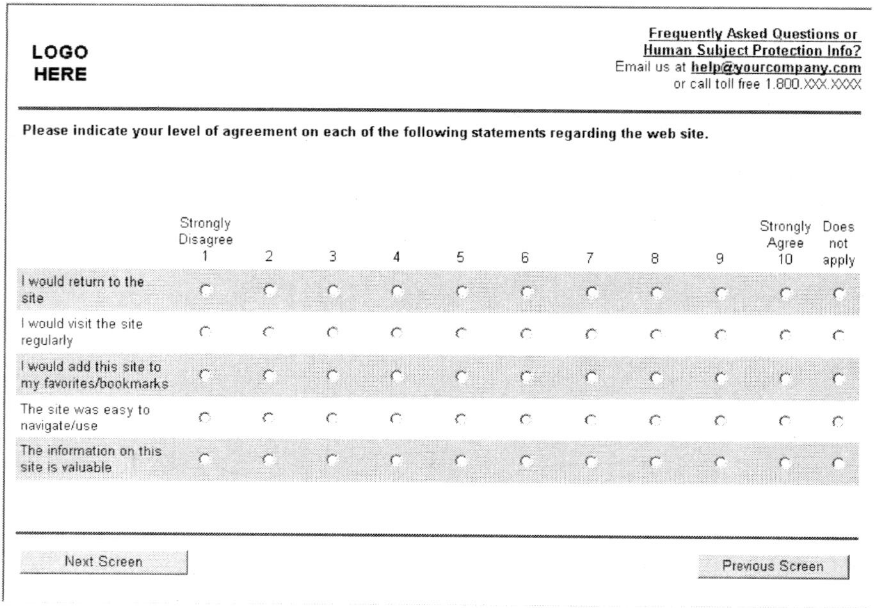

tion columns across the screen. This has been shown in at least one experimental design to impact the response provided (Tourangeau et al., 2003). In a question with a seven-point scale, displayed horizontally, one version had all response options evenly distributed across the width of the screen and a second version had response options closer to each other on the left, and more separated on the right. In the first version, the visual midpoint was at the fourth option (which is the conceptual midpoint for the response options provided). In the second version, the visual midpoint was closer to the fifth option. The result was that they found significantly higher responses in the treatment in the second version.

A grid question should be presented such that all components of the grid fit within one browser screen. If scrolling is required because of the height of the grid, they should not be allowed to require scrolling so far that the column/response headers fall off the top of the visible browser screen. If this occurs, and keeping the grid on one page is still required, then some design for creating a second row of column headers that will be available should be used. A solution could include creating a new grid question on the same page or creating column footers (mirroring the headers) attached to the bottom of the grid. To improve readability of grid question rows, use a light gray background shade for alternating rows. HTML Red-Green-Blue (RRGGBB) color code #CCCCCC is the best shading color to maximize contrast with black text across different browsers and operating systems. Other shades of gray may look fine in some browsers, but may appear much darker with different browsers, ultimately reducing the readability of the text for some respondents.

Grid questions should only be used when single choice response options are required, with each question presented as a row in the grid. Multi-response questions should not be included in grid questions, as they have caused considerable confusion with respondents not understanding the task. While we have no empirical evidence to show any data quality issues with regards to the use of multi-response questions within a grid, we do have ample reports from the technical support specialists that such question design is problematic with respondents. It is also important to avoid using grid questions that are designed with the column header containing the question and the rows containing the responses. Considerable confusion arises with this design, as respondents frequently don't notice format and attempt to respond to questions by row. Further discussion of the application of this standard can be found later in this article.

Respondent Input/Response Formats

Standard HTML provides more than enough standard form elements that can be used to collect all different kinds of Web-based survey responses. Standards that guide their use focus on consistency of use, not only from one Web-based survey to another, but also with standard means for collecting other kinds of user input on the Web, such as is done in most e-commerce functions.

For single response questions, radio buttons should be used for respondent input. For categorical multiple response option questions, check boxes should be used. Drop-down boxes may be used only for single response options with more than about eight codes in which the respondent is likely to know the answer without having to view the full list. Questions where the responses included state, country, or month are good examples of questions that can be presented in drop-down boxes. Drop-down box should not be preloaded with an answer.

Generally, do not use list boxes for most multiple response option questions. Only use list boxes when the list of responses exceeds twenty and the question is one that the respondent is likely to know the answer to prior to viewing the response options.

Experiments conducted by Couper et al. (2003) provide the empirical support for the set of standards around categorical response option questions. They found support for theories of "satisficing," where respondents select the option that takes the least amount of cognitive effort to select, and they coin the term "visibility principal." They find that respondents will be more likely to select responses that are visible without additional effort. This principal essentially calls into question any format other than radio buttons and check boxes for categorical responses, as all other possible formats (pull-down lists and list boxes) may increase the "satisficing" effects found in the survey data.

Questions that require numeric or short text response options should utilize the text HTML form field. The field should be spaced to provide enough width to accommodate the expected response, but no wider than necessary. Couper et al. (2001) found a significantly higher proportion of invalid responses when respondents were randomly provided with a long (wide) text box over a short (narrow) text box in which the expected response was to be a number between zero and ten. The long box prompted respondents to provide long text or range responses rather than single numeric values.

For questions requiring potentially long written responses, the HTML memo form field should be used. Memo fields should be spaced to fit approximately sixty columns wide and between five and ten columns high. If possible, memo fields should be set to allow word wrapping and should not contain any limitation on text length.

Survey Navigation/Interaction

Navigation through the survey should be consistent throughout the survey and should be based upon action buttons that are different than any response input element. For survey navigation, a "next screen" or "next question" button should be displayed on all pages. The next screen button should be placed in the lower left corner of the screen. If it is desired that the respondent be allowed to back up to previous questions, then a "previous screen" or "previous question" button should be displayed. The placement of this button should be in the bottom right corner of the visible browser screen. See Figures 1-3 for acceptable use and placement of navigation buttons. Empirical evidence for this design is currently weak; several pilot studies conducted at MSIResearch have failed to demonstrate any significant effect of the button placement.

However, such studies have been conducted with populations that could be considered *professional respondents* as they were members of Web-based panels who have signed up to participate in Web-based surveys. These respondents may be less susceptible to poor designs in Web-based surveys than more general populations.

The theoretical framework for this standard, however, has three key components that make it a compelling design. First, as described by Tourangeau et al. (2003), a visual "left and top mean first" heuristic may exist and may be interpreted to impact the placement of on-screen navigation items such that they fall where the respondent spends most of his/her time viewing the survey page. Placing the appropriate button to continue in the survey on the left may bring the action closer to the respondents' "left and top" visual field. Similarly, most Web-based surveys provide questions and responses that are left justified.[1] Thus, placing the "next" button on the left side of the screen will facilitate its use. And lastly, a technical issue with how most Web-based survey systems interface with HTML may clinch the reason for a left placement of a "next" button. Web browsers will automatically "focus" the use of the "Enter" or "Return" keyboard key on the next available HTML form button. When responding to the survey, if a respondent clicks their response, then taps the "Enter" key on their keyboard, the button that will activate will be the button that is closest to the top left corner of the browser screen. Placing the "Previous" button on the left would theoretically lead to a higher number of respondents accidentally backing up in the survey. In some situations, this technical limitation can be overcome; however, many Web-based survey software systems do not provide the ability to control the focus of the buttons on the screen, and even if they do, some Web browsers are not compatible with this capability.

Various sources in the Web site usability literature support this design. In their book on Web site design, Nielsen and Tahir (2002) strongly recommend that all Web site navigation should utilize buttons across the top of the page, down the left side of the page, or listed as categories in the middle of the page content. Given that survey navigation needs to be separated from the question and responses on the page, the last suggestion is not very practical in Web-based survey design. Because we propose other content to be placed at the top of the screen, it may not be very feasible within our standards. It would also violate another recommendation by Nielsen and Tahir that navigation should not be placed in or around any "banner" areas such as we have designed in these standards to be presented across the top of the screen. Placing the most used navigation component on the left side of the screen, close to the primary content of the page (the question and answer in our application) fits theories of good Web site design.

The most common critique we hear of our standard for placing the "next" button on the left side of the screen is that it is counterintuitive to those who like their Web-based surveys to emulate paper surveys, with the function of flipping to the next page completed by turning the page from the lower right corner of the survey. While no specific research has been found that explores how this may impact survey completion or data quality, we can point to an article by Nielsen (1998) where he describes usability issues with electronic books. He declares that "page turning remains a bad interface," and describes how users quickly forget about any screen to paper metaphor after they learn the interface that is provided.

While the "quit survey" button is offered standard in most Web-based survey software systems, researchers should not offer the respondent an additional way to leave the survey. Respondents are always able to quit the survey by simply closing their browser. Survey systems should be saving the responses at each screen, so the use of such a button is not necessary.

Validations can be used for respondent authentication, data type and format checks, range checks, consistency checks, and complex computations (Peytchev & Crawford, 2003). Validations that enforce required responses should be used on all closed-ended response. The ideal implementation of this standard is by using what Peytchev and Crawford term a "soft prompt." Soft prompts use an error message to inform the respondent that they had not provided a response to the question, and provides them with the opportunity to do so, to continue without further response, or to explain their lack of response. The quality benefits of this approach are currently unknown, but the costs for implementation are large (due to the much more complex programming instructions required). So, we feel an adequate standard for now is if such questions require responses to proceed, but offer a reserved (opt-out) code such as "Rather not say," "Don't know," or "Not applicable." Open-end questions should not contain required response validations.

If validations are utilized, error messages triggered by validations should be clearly written, consistently applied, and placed in red text immediately below the question.

Application to Community-Based Research

Using the design standards outlined in this chapter, we have piloted and conducted several Web-based surveys in a variety of school-based settings within the past two years, and we would like to highlight some practical experiences to assist other researchers. Web-based surveys were conducted as part of prevention activities to assist middle schools, high schools and colleges evaluate the extent of violence, alcohol and other drug use (Boyd et al., 2003; McCabe et al., 2003; McCabe et al., 2002).

In one set of studies, our aim was to examine the feasibility of implementing a Web-based survey approach for collecting data in a racially and economically diverse public school district in the midwestern United States during the spring of 2002. The survey questions and implementation schedule was consistent with national school-based surveys regarding alcohol and other drug use (Fendrich & Johnson, 2001; Johnston et al., 2002). The Web-based survey was fielded using computer labs available within each school. A coordinated community-based approach that involved researchers, community members, school district personnel, and teachers was implemented to complete the survey effort.

The Web-based survey instrument was programmed using an earlier version of the standards contained within this article. During the survey data collection, we were present in the same room as the students and actively fielded usability related questions that came up. We also reviewed the collected data for patterns that would identify problems in our standards. For the purpose of this article, we will focus on how our standards fared in this school-based survey.

Most significantly, the data collection effort achieved an overall response rate of 89 percent, including absentees and refusals, for students in 6th through 11th grade. In particular, completed questionnaires were obtained from 92 percent of students in sixth grade, 95 percent of students in seventh grade, and 96 percent of students in eighth grade, which reflect better-than-average response rates, compared to similar age groups from other school-based alcohol and other drug studies (e.g., Johnston et al., 2002). Consistent with most school-based research, absentees constituted nearly all of the non-respondents in the present study (Johnston et al., 2002). More specifically, approximately 7 percent of the entire sample (n = 117) was absent during the administration of the Web survey in the middle and high schools. Our findings were also in line with national studies in that less than one percent of students (n = 19) had a parent refuse participation in the study (Johnston et al., 2002).

Most notably, there were no racial differences in the response rates between White (88 percent) and African American (91 percent) students in the district. African American students were equally as likely to complete once they started the survey. Overall, these findings bode well for using Web-based approaches in racially and economically diverse school districts.

Furthermore, this experience demonstrated how the Web-based screen design standards could effectively be applied to a community-based research design with positive results and high quality data. No questions were found to have disproportionately higher levels of missing data, there were very few break-offs, and respondents generally reported that they enjoyed the survey-taking experience to the survey administrators present in the room during administration. In the end, there were no horror stories to tell of this data collection experience. However, this is not to say that lessons were not learned, leading to improved standards for future studies.

In this pilot study, we learned valuable lessons about the design of grid questions. In every group of approximately 30 students taking the survey at the same time, we experienced a handful of students who reported problems progressing past a question asking how they travel to and from school each day.[2]

The question asked respondents to select one response in each row. As shown in Figure 6, we used an instruction to "Choose one answer for each column." We also provided shading to group the column responses together. The previous eight questions asked in this survey were all grid questions formatted such that each question was in a row rather than a

FIGURE 6. A Problematic Grid Question Design

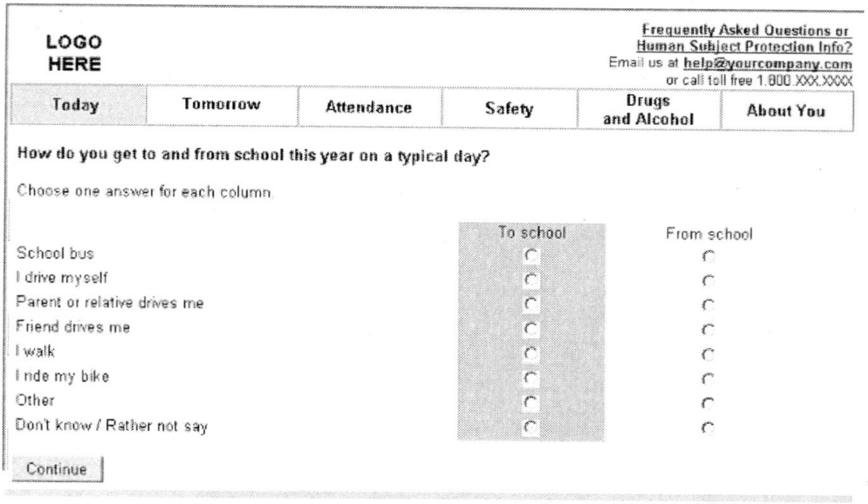

column. Even with the clear instructions and shading change, respondents struggled with this question, first attempting to respond to each row. One common question was "What if I take the bus *to* and *from* school?" This demonstrated to us that respondents were assuming that they could only provide one answer in each row. Then, many who did provide a response in both columns would then ask, "The survey won't allow me to continue without answering in each row, but the buttons only allow me to respond once in each column." Because most questions in this survey were "forced" responses where a substantive or opt-out response "don't know/rather not say" was required for the respondent to continue in the survey, the respondents were *assuming* that this one was also forced (it was), but rather than trying to submit their responses with one selection in each column (which would have been a valid response), they became frustrated and claimed they could not proceed. In several instances, the authors noted that respondents simply tried clicking on several responses, apparently without regard to the substance of the question, before finally trying (and succeeding) to continue by selecting the "Continue" button. As we were overwhelmed with trouble on this question, as administrators of the survey, we began to make announcements to clarify how this question functioned once the first student in each group arrived at this question. The announcement reduced the confusion and subsequent questions. This experience was validated by our technical support specialists who also reported similar troubles on similarly designed questions in other surveys of different populations. From these difficulties emerged the standards detailed in this paper about grid questions.

Evaluating a past survey with the hindsight of knowledge gained as new standards develop demonstrated how easy it is to blindly make errors in design that could have impacted data quality. In writing this article, the authors reviewed screenshots of the full pilot study and found at least one occasion where a current standard (not in place at the time of this survey) was violated. It is unknown if such violations may have impacted the quality of the data because no experimental comparison exists to provide a benchmark for any difference. The one violation noted is shown in Figure 7. The response columns were formatted in a manner (closer together on the left and further apart on the right) that is consistent with the treatment in the Tourangeau et al. (2003) experiment discussed earlier in this article that resulted in a shift of substantive responses. Given this finding, we have made note of this potential problem for any future analysis using the responses gathered by this question.

FIGURE 7. A Violation of the Column with Standard

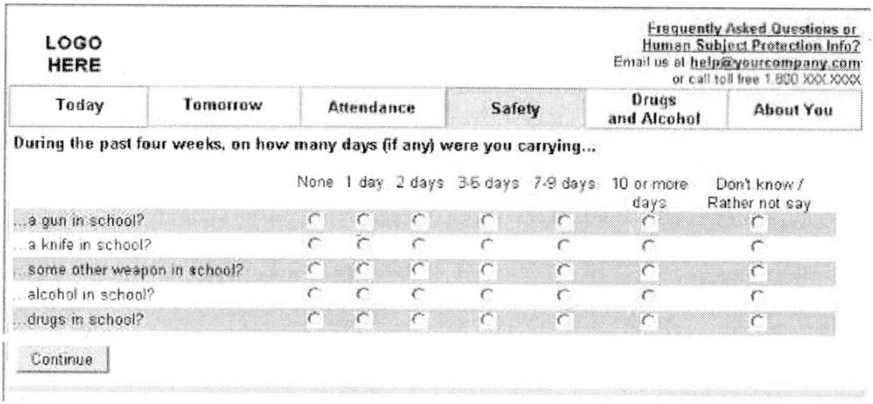

In a second study, the authors surveyed a college-based population to examine whether our standards applied to Web-based surveys could allow us to collect representative data with similar substantive responses as compared to more traditional U.S. mail approaches. The authors compared the use of a Web-based survey and hardcopy mailed survey on a college campus (McCabe et al., 2002). We found no significant differences in the distributions of race, class year and age between the samples obtained by the two survey modes.

Past research has shown that data collection modality can lead to substantially different prevalence estimates regarding illicit drug use among adolescents and young adults (e.g., Fendrich & Johnson, 2001; Sudman, 2001; Turner et al., 1998; Wright et al., 1998). Past research has also found racial differences in survey mode effects, and we wanted to examine whether the standard Web-based survey produced similar mode effects across additional racial/ethnic categories (Aquilino, 1994). Equivalent alcohol and other drug questionnaire items were compared to determine whether the U.S. mail or Web distributions were significantly different as a function of race/ethnicity. We found that there were no significant substantive differences found between the alcohol and other drug use variables (McCabe et al., 2002). This finding provides further support for minimal substantive differences in the prevalence estimates of alcohol and other drug use between Web-based and mail surveys (Bason, 2000; Miller et al., 2002).

Like the middle and high school experience, applying the Web-based survey design standards to a distributed[3] study of college students continued to demonstrate that with a well-designed Web-based survey, the Web mode can prove to be a viable means for collecting survey data. No significant design standard was changed by this study. We view this study as a significant validation of the current standards, as they were shown to produce comparable, if not improved, data quality to other, more traditional, self-administered data collection modes.

CONCLUSION/FUTURE DIRECTIONS

Web-based surveys are becoming an everyday tool for many researchers and evaluators. As with other new modes of data collection, there will continue to be a period where many researchers will conduct Web-based surveys with little regard to the impact those designs are having on total survey error.[4] Until recently, most Web-based designs have been driven by Web programmer creativity or software capability. As standards are developed and perfected, it is hoped that software developers will shift their focus to facilitate researchers' need to develop Web-based surveys that meet the standards.

Based on our research experiences, there are several implications for future work and research in the area of prevention and intervention. First, it would be helpful for prevention and intervention researchers' to describe the screen design of their Web-based surveys to allow for comparisons to be made between studies. As illustrated in this chapter, one possibility would be to include actual screen shots of key questions used in studies when reporting results. Second, it is important to know what types of screen design formats cause problems for respondents so other researchers can avoid making the same mistakes. Third, it is critical to examine how substantive responses compare between well-designed Web-based surveys and other survey modes. Additionally, it is equally important to examine how different screen design formats within Web-based surveys impact substantive responses. Finally, it will be important to monitor the efficacy of Web-based surveys across different sub-populations. The majority of our examples came from adolescent and young adult school-based student populations, and it is very possible that Web-based surveys are less effective with different age groups and individuals with lower levels of computer literacy.

In conclusion, we can comfortably say that when a well thought through standard for Web-based survey design is employed, the result can be a high quality data collection. However, it is also clear that more work needs to be done to continue the improvement of Web-based survey design standards as the technology and methods mature.

We hope that this article will provide researchers who are interested in the improvement of Web-based survey designs to validate or refute the standards presented. Although we only focused on screen design issues, we also encourage the development of standards for Web-based questionnaire writing, respondent communications, and data collection processes that were not discussed in this article. It will be through such scientific collaboration and exploration that as survey researchers, our collective efforts will provide a platform on which future data collections may be conducted with full assurances of quality data.

NOTES

1. Bowker and Dillman (2000) demonstrated inconclusive results when comparing left and right justification in a Web-based survey, but left justification is clearly the standard design provided by all Web-based survey software systems; thus, by default it has become the unwritten standard among Web-based survey research designers. While we see no evidence that suggests a change may be required, it would be useful to have data to support this basic premise of Web-based survey design.

2. We have included a screenshot of the question in Figure 6, as it was presented in this study, not only to show how this question helped us improve our standards, but also to demonstrate how standards evolve over time. This survey was designed using standards current to MSIResearch in late 2001. To protect the identity of the school district involved in this study, small edits have been made to the question in this figure, as well as Figure 7, to mask the district name.

3. We label this study "distributed" in that the survey invitations were e-mailed and each respondent was on their own in responding. This data collection approach does not benefit from the ability of the researchers to be physically present during the survey taking. We rely completely on respondent reports through the technical support specialists as well as evaluation of respondent data to tell us of problematic designs.

4. See Groves, 1989, for a thorough discussion of "total survey error."

REFERENCES

Aquilino, W.S. 1994. "Interview mode effects in surveys of drug and alcohol use: A field experiment." *Public Opinion Quarterly* 58: 210-240.

Baker, R.P., Crawford, S., & Swinehart, J. 2002. "Development and testing of Web questionnaires." Forthcoming Monograph from the 2002 International Conference on Questionnaire Development, Evaluation, and Testing Methods, Charleston, SC.

Bason, J.J. 2000. "Comparison of telephone, mail, Web, and IVR surveys of drug and alcohol use among university of Georgia students." Paper presented at the Annual Meeting of the American Association of Public Opinion Research, Portland, Oregon.

Benway, J.P. 1998. "Banner blindness: The irony of attention grabbing on the World Wide Web." Proceedings of the Human Factors and Ergonomics Society 42nd Annual Meeting, 1, 463-467.

Bowker, D., & Dillman, D.A. 2000. "An experimental evaluation of left and right oriented screens for Web questionnaires." Retrieved July 26, 2003, from *http://survey.sesrc.wsu.edu/dillman/papers/AAPORpaper00.pdf*.

Boyd, C.J., Teter, C.J., & McCabe, S.E. 2003. "The abuse of asthma inhalers by middle and high school students." Forthcoming in the *Journal of Adolescent Health*.

Conrad, F., Couper, M.P., Rourangeau, R., & Peytchev, A. 2003. "Effectiveness of progress indicators in Web-based surveys: It's what's up front that counts." Paper presented at the 4th ASC International Conference on Survey & Statistical Computing. Warwick University, September.

Couper, M.P. 2000. "Web-based surveys: A review of issues and approaches." *Public Opinion Quarterly*, Vol. 64, No. 4, Winter: 464-494.

Couper, M.P., Traugott, M.W., & Lamias, M.J. 2001. "Web survey design and administration." *Public Opinion Quarterly* 65: 230-253.

Couper, M.P., & Hansen, S. E. 2002. "Computer-assisted interviewing." In *Handbook of Interview Research: Context & Method*. Eds. Gubrium, J.F. and Holstein, J.A. Sage, Thousand Oaks.

Couper, M.P., Tourangeau, R., Conrad, F., Crawford, S. 2003. "What they see is what we get: Response options for Web-based surveys." *Social Science Computer Review*. Vol. 31, No. 4, Winter.

Crawford, S., Couper, M., & Lamias, M. 2000. "Web-based surveys: Perceptions of burden." *Social Science Computer Review*. Vol. 19, No. 2, Summer: 146-162.

Crawford, S., McCabe, S., Couper, M.P., & Boyd, C. 2002. "From mail to Web: Improving response rates and data collection efficiencies." Paper presented at the ICIS 2002-International Conference on Improving Surveys. Copenhagen, Denmark, August 25-28.

Dillman, D. 2000. *Mail and Internet Surveys: The Tailored Design Method*. Wiley, New York.

Dillman D.A., Tortora, R.D., Bowker, D. 1998. "Principals for constructing Web-based surveys." Retrieved December 21, 1999, from *http://survey.sesrc.wsu.edu/dillman/papers/Websurveyppr.pdf*.

Fendrich, M. & Johnson, T.P. 2001. "Examining prevalence differences in three national surveys of youth: Impact of consent procedures, mode and editing rules." *Journal of Drug Issues* 31: 615-642.

Groves, R.M. 1989. *Survey Errors and Survey Costs*. Wiley, New York.

Groves, R.M., Beimer, P., Lyberg, L.E., Massey, J.T., Nicholls II, W.L., & Waksberg, J. 1988. *Telephone Survey Methodology*. Wiley, New York.

Horrigan, J.B., & Rainie, L. 2002. "The broadband difference." Retrieved July 26, 2003, from *http://www.pewinternet.org/reports/pdfs/PIP_Broadband_Report.pdf*.

Johnston, L.D., O'Malley, P.M., & Bachman, J.G. 2002. "Monitoring the future national survey results on drug use." Volume I: Secondary School Students. Bethesda, MD: National Institute on Drug Abuse.

McCabe, S.E., Boyd, C.J., Couper, M.P., Crawford, S., & d'Arcy, H. 2002. "Mode effects for collecting alcohol and other drug use data: Web and U.S. mail." *Journal of Studies on Alcohol* 63(6): 755-761.

McCabe, S.E., Teter, C.J., & Boyd, C.J. 2003. "The use, misuse and diversion of prescription stimulants among middle and high school students." Forthcoming in *Substance Use and Misuse*.

Miller, E.T., Neal, D.J., Roberts, L.J., Baer, J.S., Cressler, S.O., Metrik, J., & Marlatt, G.A. 2002. "Test-retest reliability of alcohol measures: Is there a difference between internet-based assessment and traditional methods?" *Psychology of Addictive Behaviors* 16: 56-63.

Nielsen, J. 2000. *Designing Web Usability*. New Riders Publishing, Indianapolis.

Nielsen, J. & Tahir, M. 2002. *Homepage Usability*. New Riders Publishing, Indianapolis.

Pealer, L., Weiler, R.M., Pigg, R.M., Miller, D., & Dorman, S.M. 2001. "The feasibility of a Web-based surveillance system to collect health risk behavior data from college students." *Health Education & Behavior* 28: 547-171-179.

Peytchev, A., & Crawford, S. 2003. "Real-time validations in Web-based Surveys." Paper presented at the 2003 Annual Meeting of the Association for Public Opinion Research. Nashville, TN. May.

Standard and Poor's. 2002. "School evaluation services." Accessed: *http://www.ses. standardandpoors.com/*.

Sudman, S. 2001. "Examining substance abuse data collection methodologies." *Journal of Drug Issues* 31: 695-716.

Tourangeau, R., Couper, M.P., & Conrad, F. 2003. "The impact of the visible: Images, spacing, and other visual cues in Web-based surveys." Paper presented at the WSS/FCSM Seminar on the Funding Opportunity in Survey Methodology. May 22.

Turner, C.F., Ku, L., Rogers, S.M., Lindberg, L.D., Pleck, J.H., & Sonenstein, F.L. 1998. "Adolescent sexual behavior, drug use, and violence: Increased reporting with computer survey technology." *Science* 280: 867-873.

Vehovar, V., Lozar Manfreda, K., and Batagelj, Z. 2001. "Errors in Web-based surveys." E-Proceedings of the 53rd Session of the ISI, Seoul, South Korea, August 22-29.

Wright, D.L., Aquilino, W.S., & Supple, A.I. 1998. "A comparison of computer-assisted and paper-and-pencil self-administered questionnaires in a survey on smoking, alcohol, and other drug use." *Public Opinion Quarterly* 62: 331-353.

Assessing Quality Assurance
of Self-Help Sites on the Internet

Steven Godin
Jack Truschel
Vasu Singh

East Stroudsburg University

SUMMARY. One of the most common uses of the Internet is to access health and mental health information. While thousands of Websites have been developed to provide consumers with health and mental health information, little has been done regarding assuring the quality of the material provided. This article presents the quality assurance assessment findings of 80 Websites that provide consumers information on common DSM-IV psychiatric disorders. The results of this assessment found a number of concerns: (1) a lack of evidence of qualified authors; (2) a lack of any formal review, or existence of a review board; (3) a lack of timely updating of the Website material; (4) potential conflicts of interest with advertisements; (5) average readability indexes at the 11.2 grade reading level; and (6) a paucity of Websites that use any evidence of behavior change theories. The authors recommend a standards be established to assure quality of the self-help information provided on the Internet. Furthermore, the au-

---

Address correspondence to: Steven Godin, Community Health Education Program, East Stroudsburg University, 200 Prospect Street, East Stroudsburg, PA 18301.

[Haworth co-indexing entry note]: "Assessing Quality Assurance of Self-Help Sites on the Internet." Godin, Steven, Jack Truschel, and Vasu Singh. Co-published simultaneously in *Journal of Prevention & Intervention in the Community* (The Haworth Press, Inc.) Vol. 29, No. 1/2, 2005, pp. 67-84; and: *Technology Applications in Prevention* (ed: Steven Godin) The Haworth Press, Inc., 2005, pp. 67-84. Single or multiple copies of this article are available for a fee from The Haworth Document Delivery Service [1-800-HAWORTH, 9:00 a.m. - 5:00 p.m. (EST). E-mail address: docdelivery@haworthpress.com].

http://www.haworthpress.com/web/JPIC
Digital Object Identifier: 10.1300/J005v29n01_05

thors encourage future Web-based self-help efforts to apply the embedded power of the Internet to offer interactive, theory-driven educational interventions to not only improve knowledge, but also behavior. *[Article copies available for a fee from The Haworth Document Delivery Service: 1-800-HAWORTH. E-mail address: <docdelivery@haworthpress.com> Website: <http://www.HaworthPress.com> © 2005 by The Haworth Press, Inc. All rights reserved.]*

KEYWORDS. Self-help, Internet, quality-assurance, health-literacy, psychoeducation

INTRODUCTION

In this article, the authors first describe the rapid adoption of the Internet by consumers within the U.S. and abroad. A review of literature is provided on how frequently Internet health Websites are used in our society. However, despite consumers' use of Internet health sites, many find the health information not trustworthy, nor of high quality. The authors describe the construction of a quality assurance tool that can be used to assess Internet health sites, and demonstrate its use in assessing 80 self-help Websites for common mental health problems. The results indicate that significant changes are needed in the design and delivery of self-help sites on the Internet. Last, the authors project into the future how the landscape of Internet health will change with the Web playing an important role in prevention and tertiary service delivery.

THE DIFFUSION OF INTERNET USE TO ACCESS HEALTH INFORMATION

The adoption of the Internet by consumers has occurred faster than any other mass media venue introduced in the United States including the radio and television. The adoption curve of the Internet has been staggering, with 26% of the U.S. population having Internet access at home or in the workplace in 1998, and increasing to 60% (i.e., 169 million residents) in 2001 (U.S. Dept. of Commerce; Nielsen/NetRatings, 2001. As of 2000, the Internet ranked fourth in usage rates of consumer media. Over the last five years, the majority of the Internet users in the

U.S. report annual household incomes over $75,000, sparking concerns about a great "digital divide." However, the increasing rates of Internet adoption have gradually slowed in higher income groups (due to market saturation); whereas the rates of adoption in lower income households now represent the fastest growing segment in the population (National Telecommunications & Information Administration, 2000; Nie & Ebring, 2000). Diffusion of Internet access is also expanding globally. Recently, it was estimated that over 400 million people worldwide were using the Internet in 2000, with this number expected to rise considerably in the next decade (NUA, 2000).

People go online for a variety of reasons. While many use the Internet to communicate via chat rooms (21%), or send/receive e-mails (89%), the primary reason is to gather information (95%) (NUA, 2000). Of all topic areas of searched, obtaining preventive information about health was one of the most common. In 2000, 86% of adults used the Internet to access health information (Harris Interactive, 2000; Pew Internet & American Life Project, 2000). The Internet has been responsive to the demand for health information. While the actual number of health-related Websites is unknown, it was estimated that the more than 19,000 sites recently indexed in a search using Yahoo in spring 2001 may only represent a small portion of the total number of health-related Websites that actually exist (Robert Wood Johnson Foundation, 2001).

The public seeks information on a variety of health topics. People like using the Web for seeking health information because of the quick and convenient access to information, while maintaining the feeling of privacy (Risk & Petersen, 2002). According to the Symposium on E-Healthcare Strategies (2000), users were reported to search the Internet most for health and mental health information. Table 1 provides a rank ordering of the diseases or health conditions that were most commonly searched in the late 1990s.

TABLE 1. Most Commonly Searched Health and Mental Health Topics

1) Depression	6) Hypertension
2) Allergies/Sinus Conditions	7) Migraines
3) Cancer	8) Anxiety
4) Bipolar Disorder	9) CVD/Heart Disease
5) Arthritis/Rheumatism	10) Sleep Disorders

CONCERNS ABOUT THE QUALITY
OF HEALTH INFORMATION ON THE WEB

While a growing number of people may use the Internet to access health information, many are also concerned about the accuracy of information they receive. In one review of the literature, McLeod (1998) references a number of studies that have demonstrated that many Internet sites provide the public with incomplete, inaccurate, and sometimes misleading health information. Other researchers have shown that the quality of Internet health sites varies considerably, with some sites being excellent, and others being poorly designed, or providing dangerous false information written by individuals with little or no professional training in the health field (Berland et al., 2001; Craige et al., 2002; Eysenbach, Powell, & Kuss, 2002; & Crocco, Villasis-Keever, & Jadad, 2002). In a popular opinion poll by *Prevention Magazine* (1998), 64% of Web users had little or no trust in the accuracy of Internet-provided health information.

Pergament (1999) reports that when consumers access Internet health sites, some are able to comprehend the material, while others misinterpret the information, or are led to believe they may have conditions or health needs that do not exist. The average grade level of narrative provided on health Websites often exceeds that of the user. In one study, the average readability index for health sites was at the collegiate level (Robinson et al., 1998). However, it appears that the Internet is not the only source of misinformation, inaccuracies, and poorly designed health information. A number of studies remind us that the problems witnessed regarding quality of health information on the Internet have also been long-standing with traditional print media (Payne et al., 1998; Slaytor & Ward, 1998; Smith et al., 1998) (all in Risk, 2002). Risk (2002) simply states that the Internet has become a new delivery system for providing health information; the health profession continues to make the same mistakes it has always made whether it be with the Internet or traditional print media.

EFFORTS TO ASSURE QUALITY
OF HEALTH INFORMATION SITES ON THE INTERNET

In order to protect the public, many believe there is a significant need to harness Web-based health material and oversee the quality of health information provided to the public. There are a variety of avenues one can take to ensure quality of health information provided on the Internet. Some suggest that accrediting bodies such as the American Accreditation Healthcare Commission (URAC), the National Committee for Quality Assurance (NCQA), the Food and Drug Administration (FDA), or the Joint Commission on Accreditation of Healthcare Organizations (JCAHO) should take a leadership role in the accreditation of health Websites. However, given the global nature of the Web, many believe it would be difficult and burdensome to accredit Websites managed outside the U.S. As an alternative, others recommend utilization of a "rating system," or using a "consumers' report" model for recommending specific sites that adhere to various criteria including accuracy of health information.

Some believe that a rating system should transcend beyond just looking at health information accuracy, but also include a variety of other criteria that can improve quality. Jadad and Gagliardi (1998), suggested that all health Websites should have a basic set of criteria including: (1) Name, affiliation, credentials of the author(s)/creators of the Website; (2) References/citations to support any health information narrative; (3) Acknowledgment of any perceived or real conflict of interest; and (4) Providing information on the date of most recent update.

To summarize the above paragraph, by including the name, affiliation, and credentials of the authors or creators of the site, one can ascertain whether the site is maintained, or authored by someone who has the appropriate professional qualifications for the educational material provided. Referencing or providing citations can be useful in supporting any factual information, claims or recommendations provided by the author(s). Since Websites are financially supported in a variety of ways, acknowledging potential conflicts of interest (i.e., recommending a product that the site is selling, or receiving commissions on) can be helpful to consumers. Given the ongoing advances routinely made in preventive care and health services, indicating when the Website was most recently updated would help the visitor determine whether the information on the site is current or outdated.

Health on the Net Foundation, which was created in 1995, developed a "Health Code of Conduct" called "HON" as a quality assurance mechanism. Hersch (1999), and more recently, Dorman (2002), report that sites that adhere to the HON code would be allowed to display the "HON seal of approval." Those sites with this approval would provide the following: (1) Professionally qualified authors for narrative written within the site; (2) A statement stating the site is designed to support, not replace, professional services; (3) Confidentiality of the visitor's identity is secured; (4) Educational material is referenced, with referral to other Websites (via links) when available; (5) All claims and benefits reported within the site must be supported by evidence and referenced; (6) The site must provide contact information and e-mail addresses for visitors to be able to ask further questions, and have these questions answered in a timely fashion; (7) The site must provide information about the financial support for the Website; (8) The site must indicate whether advertising within the site is a source of funding; and if so, (9) The site must keep advertising information separate from the main body of health information provided.

To summarize the above, by providing authorship information site visitors will be able to know whether the health information is written by a qualified professional. Furthermore, the trustworthiness of material is improved by referencing information, as well as claims and benefits cited. Visitors are provided further information by visiting links to other Websites, or by having the opportunity to e-mail the author(s) to have their questions answered. To alleviate liability issues, many experts recommend that approved sites provide a "disclaimer statement" that indicates the Website material is "population-based" or generic educational material that augments, but does not replace, professional services. Confidentiality issues regarding visits to health Websites has been a significant concern for those using the Internet. Many Websites that are visited by the public attach "cookies" to the user's hard drive to track the Web movements, and amount of time spent within a given Website. Most of the time, this information is used for marketing research and for advertising products to the user. However, the use of cookies can lead to abuse. For example, let's say a company employee during the lunch break visits a Website to learn more about depression and coping strategies. When this employee returns to the company home page, the company (through the use of cookies) will have information about the Websites that employee visited during that lunch break and future ones. If a supervisor is made aware of the various visits an employee made to a Website that helps people cope with depression, would this knowledge impact decisions regarding future promotions of the given employee?

Finally, conflicts of interest need to be addressed. Many sites receive financial support through advertising products and/or services. For example, let's say a consumer is visiting a Website on depression to gather information on effective coping. During the browse, a pharmaceutical company has an attractive, blinking advertisement stating "use product X to relieve your symptoms of depression." When the consumer clicks on this ad, he/she lands within the pharmaceutical site which encourages the consumer to consider using the medication. In turn, the referring Website (i.e., the depression education site) receives commission reimbursement from the drug company. If the depression education site relies on these commissions for longevity, there may be a conflict of interest. In some cases, advertisements are so subtle that the consumer is unaware they have left the original site visited and are now receiving educational material elsewhere from the drug company. This is especially the case when advertisements are embedded within the educational text, and/or not in a separate section of the Webpage.

Ling (1999) and Kim (1999) also published a series of similar guidelines to ensure quality of health-related Websites. While many of these guidelines parallel the recommendations presented above, there are a few additional contributions to assessing quality. Namely, does the Website: (1) Have a formal review process (i.e., peer reviewed, editorial board); (2) Indicate the nature of the audience the site is intended for (i.e., teens, adults, the elderly, or health care professionals); and (3) Have a design that is easy to use/navigate through?

To summarize the above, similar to the use of references and citing authorship, the use of peer review or an editorial board provides further evidence that the information comes from a trustworthy source. Many web browsers, in search of useful information find Websites that are designed for health care professionals, and not lay audiences. On the other hand, other sites have material written or presented in a way for easier comprehension (i.e., for teens or for the elderly). Making the visitor aware of who the site was designed for allows the user to make more informed choices about whether to stay within the site or leave for a Website more suited to their needs.

Previous Work Conducted by the Authors

Godin and colleagues (2000a, 2000b, 2001, 2002a, 2002b) have been involved with the development and refinement of a Internet health quality assurance assessment tool that includes many of the recommendations made by the authors cited above. In addition, this assessment tool also measures: (1) Whether the user is able to "interact" within the site either by answering questions presented to the user and receiving feedback; (2) A readability index of the educational material presented; (3) Whether the site overtly uses a "health behavior change theory" to support an intervention or Web-based interaction or activity; and

(4) Whether the Website places cookies on the user's hard drive, and if so, how many.

While previous Internet ratings conducted by Godin and colleagues included assessment of Websites in health education, disease management, mental health, self-help, and pharmaceutical sites, the development of the quality assurance tool was a work in progress. The primary flaws in the early research was employing multiple raters and poorly developed criteria in the rating of Websites which resulted in weak inter-rater reliability (i.e., Kappa scores of r = .56, and r = .63). The assessment instrument was refined based on this preliminary work to improve inter-rater agreement. For example, to assess the readability index of a given site, it was found that cutting and pasting three separate sections of the Website text and placing it into MS-Word to conduct a Flesch-Kincaid Readability Index improved reliability of the final composite score on readability. To assess cookies, the researchers found that the number of cookies attached to one's hard drive may be a function of the time spent, and the number of clicks within the Website. Furthermore, the researchers found it to be more user friendly to use the McAfee software "Guard-dog" to assess the number of cookies placed on the hard drive as opposed to using Windows, Netscape, or Explorer systems. In the Appendix, the refined instrument entitled the *"Quality Assurance Rating Tool for Internet Health Sites (Version 3)"* was used in the two assessment studies presented at conferences in 2002. In these two studies, inter-rater agreement improved (i.e., Kappa scores of r = .72, and r = .76). Furthermore, the inter-correlations on the readability of the three sections of text cut and pasted per rater also improved to a respectable r = .78, and r = .74.

THE PRESENT STUDY

The authors assessed the quality of self-help sites for the most common psychiatric problems experienced in the U.S, using the *"Quality Assurance Rating Tool for Internet Health Sites (Version 3)."* Using the results from the National Co-morbidity Survey (see Kessler et al., 1994), the following DSM-IV most commonly reported disorders were searched on the Internet: (1) ADD/ADHD; (2) Oppositional-Defiant Disorder; (3) Conduct Disorder; (4) Major Depression; (5) Dysthymic Disorder; (6) Specific Phobia; (7) Social Phobia; (8) Post Traumatic Stress Disorder; (9) Alcohol Abuse; and (10) Adjustment Disorders.

Methods

The ten most common DSM-IV disorders were listed and given to the authors of the present study. The authors generated a list of various lay-terms (i.e., "hyperactive child" for ADD/ADHD) for the 10 diagnoses that would be used to search the Internet for self-help/information-giving Websites. Keywords for each of disorders were entered into the search windows for Yahoo and Google that generated pages of Internet addresses within each search. Given that most Internet users only access the findings on the first page of their searches, the Websites assessed in this study were limited to those identified within the first 20 listings in each search. Only those Websites that clearly provided the user self-help-based education information was used in this study. In a number of cases, the same Websites were identified in the searches. In Table 2 is a listing of those Internet Websites that were assessed for quality assurance.

Each site was rated a total of two times by the three authors in late winter and early spring 2003. The composite of inter-rater agreement on all yes-no questions on the assessment tool was reasonable with Kappa = .73. Most questions on the rating tool had a high level of agreement. The question with the lowest inter-rater agreement measured whether the advertisements pose potential conflicts of interest. The reason why this question had lower agreement was due to the subjectivity of assessing "conflict of interest." The composite correlation between the raters' three text samples for the Flesch-Kincaid Readability Index was also acceptable at r = .70.

THE RESULTS

Of the 80 Websites that were assessed, 50 were ".com" sites. The remaining sites were ".org" (n = 26), ".net" (n = 2), and ".gov" (n = 2). There were no ".edu" nor ".mil" sites evaluated in this study. In Table 3 is a summary of the assessment findings.

T-test comparisons were made between the ".com" and ".org" sites regarding: (1) the average number of months that occurred since last update; (2) the average number of links per site; (3) the average readability index; and (4) the average number of cookies placed on the hard drive. There was no significant differences in the mean number of months since most recent update, the mean number of links, nor the mean readability index. However, there was a significant difference between ".com" and ".org" in the average number of cookies placed on the user's

TABLE 2. Self-Help Websites for Common Psychiatric Disorders

1. aacap.org
2. aaets.org
3. aboutourkids.org
4. add.org
5. addclinic-az-nm.com
6. adhd.com
7. adultchildren.org
8. ahealthyme.com
9. alcoholanddrugabuse.com
10. allaboutdepression.com
11. allkids.org
12. anxietynetwork.com
13. anxietyselfhelp.com
14. athealth.com
15. behavenet.com
16. behaviormanagement.org
17. bipolarworld.net
18. chadd.org
19. conductdisorders.com
20. depression.about.com
21. depressionclinic.com
22. drkoop.com
23. dr-self-help.com
24. edutechsbs.com
25. emedicine.com
26. emh.org
27. emotional-freedom.com
28. encourageconnection.com
29. expertparents.com
30. focusas.com
31. have-a-heart.com
32. healingpanic.com
33. health.org
34. health-center.com
35. healthinmind.com
36. healthyplace.com
37. ipanic.com
38. keepkidshealthy.com
39. kidshealth.org
40. klis.com
41. mentalhealth.com
42. mentalhealth.miningco.com
43. mentalhealth.org
44. mental-health-matters.com
45. mentalhelp.net
46. metamorphosis.com
47. mhsanctuary.com
48. mhselfhelp.org
49. mhsource.com
50. mindlink.org
51. mooddisordersinfo.com
52. nami.org
53. ncptsd.org
54. NewLifeLearning.com
55. nida.nih.gov
56. nimh.nih.gov
57. nmha.org
58. noah-health.org
59. onhealth.com
60. onlinesexaddict.org
61. open-mind.org
62. panicattacks.com
63. peercenter.org
64. peoplewho.org
65. psychcentral.com
66. psychejam.com
67. psychnet-uk.com
68. psychologydoc.com
69. psychologyinfo.com
70. psychologypedia.com
71. psychwww.com
72. psyweb.com
73. ptsdalliance.org
74. schizophrenia.com
75. selfgrowth.com
76. sexualrecovery.org
77. socialphobia.org
78. teenswithproblems.com
79. thepsych.com
80. undoingdepression.com

TABLE 3. Findings from the Quality Assessment of Self-Help Websites

Assessment Item	Yes	No
Is a "Name, affiliation, credentials of the author(s)" who developed the website listed? (The Website must indicate all 3 above)	30% (n = 24)	70% (n = 56)
Does the Website provide "References/citations" for the visitor to access should he/she wish to do further investigation or reading, or substantiate the Website material?	65% (n = 52)	35% (n = 28)
Does the health site provide contact information and/or mail addresses for visitors to contact should he/she have further questions (check "contact us")?	65% (n = 52)	35% (n = 28)
Perceived/real conflict of interest: Does the site provide any *advertisements*?	34% (n = 27)	66% (n = 53)
If yes, do these advertisements pose potential conflicts of interest (i.e., potential funding for the site, or linkage to other sites to spend money, etc.)?	78% (n = 21)	22% (n = 6)
If yes, does the Website keep advertising information **separate** from the main body of health information?	56% (n = 15)	44% (n = 12)
Does the health site cite financial support for the Website?	19% (n = 15)	81% (n = 65)
Does the health portal provide a "date of the most recent update"? Make sure it states–"The site has been updated," and not have just a "date-counter."	24% (n = 19)	76% (n = 61)
If yes, how old is the most recent update? **Avg = 24.8 months; SD = 23.5**		
Do the health site articles/narrative provide evidence of professionally qualified authors?	45% (n = 36)	55% (n = 44)
Does the health site provide wording stating it is "designed to support, *not replace* PCP services (Primary Care Physicians)"?	25% (n = 20)	75% (n = 60)
Does the health site provide a disclaimer stating that the health education content is "general information" and not "individualized patient information"?	32.5% (n = 26)	67.5% (n = 54)
Does the health portal indicate to the visitor that his/her "confidentiality of information is secured"?	29% (n = 23)	71% (n = 57)
Does the health site provide "links" to other useful sites?	55% (n = 44)	45% (n = 36)
If yes, how many work? **Range was from 1 to 25 links.**		
Does the health portal indicate there is a formal review process (i.e., peer reviewed, editorial board)?	5% (n = 4)	95% (n = 76)
Does the health site mention the nature of audience that the site is intended for (e.g., youth vs. professional vs. elderly)?	22.5% (n = 18)	77.5% (n = 62)
Does the health site allow for "interaction" between the Website and user?	11% (n = 9)	89% (n = 71)
The average readability index: **Avg = 11.2 grade reading level; SD = 1.53**		
Is there any evidence of **"health behavior change"** theory, or the use of health/public health theories, or other theories from related fields?	2% (n = 1)	98% (n = 79)
Does the health site "send cookies" to your hard drive?	60% (n = 48)	40% (n = 32)
If yes, how many cookies were sent in a standardized opening of three separate pages within the Website? Avg = 1.95; SD = 2.96		

hard drive. ".Com" sites averaged 2.25 cookies, and ".org" averaged .85 cookies (T = 2.09; p < .05).

DISCUSSION OF THE FINDINGS

Using the criteria recommended by a number of authors, considerable improvements are needed in the quality of self-help sites on the Web. While the majority of sites did provide references/citations, contact information, and links to other useful sites, they fell far short in all other criteria measured. The minority of sites provided information on the author(s) who developed the site, and under 50% of sites provided evidence of qualified authors for the educational information provided. Even fewer sites indicated they had a formal review of the educational information prior to posting this information on the Website. Few sites provided information on when the site was last updated. For those sites that did, the authors were surprised at the average length of time that had transpired (i.e., approximately 2 years) since last update.

Very few sites provided information about how the site is financially supported. About one-third of the sites had advertisements, and of those advertisements, the authors felt there was a potential conflict of interest in 3 out of 4 cases. Furthermore, many of these advertisements were not separated from the main body of health information, nor were they labeled as "advertisements."

Many of the sites did not provide disclaimer statements, and in those situations where sites had disclaimer statements, they were difficult to find. Close to three-fourths of the sites did not indicate to the visitor that their "confidentiality of information was secured." Over three-fourths of the sites did not mention the nature of audience the site was intended for. However, it should be noted that in many cases, especially in DSM-IV disorders seen in youth, the Websites had language that implied that they were targeted towards parents and/or caretakers.

The readability index for the 80 Websites was very high at a 11.2 grade reading level. Considering that the average reading level for the U.S. is under 9th or 10th grade (depending on the region), the reading level for these Websites are set too high. While medical and psychological terminology may inflate the index somewhat, these terms cannot account for a level of reading this high. Most popular newspapers are written at 5th to 6th grade reading level, and one of the most sophisticated newspapers–the *New York Times*–is written at the 9th grade level. In order to assure that all visitors fully comprehend the information, the sites need to provide visitors the education material at a 5th to 6th grade reading level.

The authors were interested in whether any of the self-help, education-oriented sites provided any evidence of being based in health behavior change theory. Only one site did so modestly, with reference to the transtheoretical (stages of change) model and denial of alcohol abuse. Otherwise, the remaining sites were void of any application of behavior change theory. Furthermore, few sites allowed for the visitor to engage in some type of interactive format. Simply, rather than consider the power of the Internet in teaching various skill sets (i.e., stress reduction, problem solving, cognitive reframing, etc.), most sites provided what could be considered traditional informational "print media" using a new format of the Internet.

FUTURE DIRECTIONS

The use of the Internet as a prevention and education tool is still in its infancy. Many people in this country and abroad have concerns about their health and mental health and are accessing the Internet to receive information and preventive material. Currently, there is no standardized format for how material is presented and validated for the visitor. Furthermore, current Internet sites provide mostly static print media strategies with reading levels that may be difficult for the majority of people to understand. Whether it is the development of accreditation standards or rating systems that allow for "seals of approval," health and mental health information on the Internet needs a formal quality assurance mechanism by which consumers can benefit.

Few interventionists have conceptualized the development of Websites that use the power of Web software, which could be interfaced with theory-anchored health behavior change strategies. As the technology on the Internet improves, Web-based prevention and intervention programs can become a viable venue for the prevention and management of health and mental health problems. The Websites "eatright.org" and "shapeup.org" provide recent examples of theory-driven interventions and are starting points from which the field of Web-prevention can model.

The use of password protected sites holds promise for Websites to offer consumers messages and interventions that are tailored to their needs. The ability to collect assessment data and demographic information on such sites can lead to intervention triaging with targeted health communication that is appropriate and culturally sensitive. Consumers on such sites can provide feedback to the program, and in turn, the program can adjust to meet the needs of the specific consumer. For example, the Website can assess the user's comprehension. If the user is struggling, the Website can branch into a lower reading level as it continues to offer the education/prevention material.

As the Internet moves towards broadband implementation, the integration of multimedia methodologies with an "edutainment" ideology may provide for some exciting approaches that use video-gaming technologies coupled with cognitive behavioral skill building. Website visitors in the future may be able to interface with a variety of virtual realities where they can learn to apply life skills to reduce risk behaviors. The use of real-time, video-based chat rooms could change the landscape for how social support networks are implemented and maintained to buffer the stressors encountered by consumers.

Last, the escalating costs of health care may provide an impetus for Web-based prevention. According to Levit and colleagues, health care spending in the U.S. in 1998 cost about $1.1 trillion or 13.5% of the gross domestic product (GDP). It is estimated that health care expenditures will double by 2008, reaching $2.2 trillion or 16.2% of the GDP. This trend cannot continue, and the Web will be seen as a tool to reduce the cost of health care. This will be done with the Web providing primary prevention and consumer empowerment, risk reduction skills, as well as providing disease management and chronic care services.

REFERENCES

Berland, G. K., Fonarow, G. C., Hays, R. D. et al. (2001). Health information on the Internet: Accessibility, quality, and readability in English and Spanish. *Journal of the American Medical Association*, 285, 2612-2621.

Craigie, M., Loader, B., Burrows, R. et al. (2002). Reliability of health information on the Internet: An examination of experts' ratings. *Journal of Medical Internet Research*, 4, e2.

Crocco, A. G., Villasis-Keever, M., & Jadad, A. R. (2002). Analysis of cases of harm associated with use of health information on the Internet. *Journal of the American Medical Association*, 287, 2869-2871.

Dorman, S. M. (2002). Health of the Net Foundation: Advocating for quality health information. *Journal of School Health*, 72, 86.

Eysenbach, G., Powell, J., & Kuss, O. (2002). Empirical studies assessing the quality of health information for consumers on the World Wide Web. *Journal of the American Medical Association*, 287, 2691-2700.

Godin, S., Coke, N., Daley, M., Gimenez, M., Miele, C., Rose, E., Scheffner, S. Sposito, J., & Xu, Jie (2000, November). *Development of a quality assurance rating system for Internet disease management sites.* Paper presented at the 128th Annual Meeting of the American Public Health Association, Boston.

Godin, S., Hillman, K., Boyle, L., Cullen, L., King, J., & Petersen, M. (2000, November). *Development of a quality assurance rating system for Internet health portals.* Paper presented at the 128th Annual Meeting of the American Public Health Association, Boston.

Godin, S., Homick, H., & Walsh, E. (2001 April). *Assessing quality of mental health education sites on the Internet.* Paper presented at the 72nd Annual Meeting of the Eastern Psychological Association, Washington, DC.

Godin, S., Singh, V., & Morgan, C. (2002, May). *Quality assurance of health education on major pharmaceutical Internet sites.* Paper presented at the 2002 Midyear Scientific Conference of the Society for Public Health Education, Cincinnati, OH.

Godin, S. & Truschel, J. (2002, March). *Assessing quality of self-help education sites on the Internet.* Paper presented at the 73nd Annual Meeting of the Eastern Psychological Association, Boston.

Harris Interactive. *Explosive growth of "Cyberchondriacs" continues.* New York: NY, Harris Interactive.

Hersh, W. (1999). The quality of information on the World Wide Web. *Journal of the American College of Dentists, 66,* 43-45.

Jadad, A. & Gagliardi, A. (1998). Rating health information on the Internet: Navigating to knowledge or to Babel. *Journal of the American Medical Association, 279,* 611-614.

Kessler, R. C., McGonagle, K. A., Zhao, S. et al. (1994). Lifetime and 12-month prevalence of DSM-IIIR psychiatric disorders in the United States. Results from the National Co-morbidity Survey. *Archives of General Psychiatry, 51,* 8-19.

Kim, P. et al. (1999). Published criteria for evaluating health related websites: A review. *British Medical Journal, 318,* 647-649.

Levit, K., Cowan, C., Lazenby, H. et al. (2000). Health spending in 1998: Signals of change. *Health Affairs, 19,* 124-132.

Ling, C. (1999). Guiding patients through the maze of drug information on the Internet. *American Journal of Health-Systems Pharmacy, 56,* 212-214.

McLeod, S. D. (1998). The quality of medical information on the Internet. *Archives of Ophthalmology, 116,* 1663-1665.

National Telecommunications and Informations Administration, Rural Utilities Service (2000). *The challenge of bringing broadband service to all Americans.* Washington, DC: National Telecommunications and Information Administration.

Nie, N. H. & Erbring, L. (2000). *Internet and society: A preliminary report.* Palo Alto, CA: Stanford Institute for the Quantitative Study of Society.

Nielsen//NetRatings (2001). *Internet penetration reaches 60 percent in the U.S.: More than 168 million people have Internet access.* New York: NY, Nielsen//NetRatings.

NUA (2000). *How many online?* Dublin, Ireland: NUA, LTD.

Payne, S., Large, S., Jarrett, N., & Turner, P. (2000). Written information given to patients and families by palliative care units. *Lancet, 355,* 1792.

Pergament, D. (1999). At the crossroads: The intersection of the Internet and clinical oncology. *Oncology*, 13, 577-581.

Pew Internet and American Life Project (2000). *The online health care revolution: How the web helps Americans take better care of themselves.* Washington, DC: Pew Research Center.

Prevention Magazine (1998). *National survey of consumer reactions to direct-to-consumer advertising.* Pp 1-30, PA: Rodale.

Risk, A. & Petersen, C. (2002). Health information on the Internet: Quality issues and international initiatives. *Journal of the American Medical Association*, 287, 2713-2715.

Robert Wood Johnson Foundation (2001). *The e-health landscape.* Princeton, NJ: Robert Wood Johnson Foundation.

Robinson, T. N., Patrick, K., Eng, T.R., et al. (1998). An evidence-based approach to interactive health communication: A challenge to medicine in the information age. *Journal of the American Medical Association*, 280, 1264-1269.

Slaytor, E. K. & Ward, J.E. (1998). How risks of breast cancer and benefits of screening are communicated to women: An analysis of 58 pamphlets. *British Medical Journal*, 317, 263-264.

Smith, H., Gooding, S., Brown, R. et al. (1998). Evaluation of readability and accuracy of information leaflets in general practice for patients with asthma. *British Medical Journal*, 317, 264-265.

U.S. Department of Commerce (2002). A nation online: How Americans are expanding their use of the Internet. Washington, DC: Economics and Statistics Administration, National Telecommunications and Informations Administration.

APPENDIX
Quality Assurance Rating Tool for Internet Health Sites (Version 3)

1) WEBSITE NAME: _____

2) Is a "Name, affiliation, credentials of the author(s)" who developed the Website listed? (The Website must indicate all 3 above)

YES NO

3) Does the Website provide "References/citations" for the visitor to access should he/she wish to do further investigation or reading, or substantiate the Website material?

YES NO

4) Does the health site provide contact information and/or mail addresses for visitors to contact should he/she have further questions (check "contact us")?

YES NO

5) A. Perceived/real conflict of interest: Does the site provide any advertisements?

YES NO

B. If yes, do these advertisements pose potential conflicts of interest (i.e., potential funding for the site, or linkage to other sites to spend money, etc.)?

YES NO N/A

C. If yes, does the Website keep advertising information **separate** from main body of health information?

YES NO N/A

6) Does the health site cite financial support for the Website?

YES NO

7) Does the health portal provide a "date of the most recent update"? Make sure it states "The site has been updated," and not have just a "date-counter."

YES NO If yes, how old is the most recent update: _____ months

8) Do the health site articles/narrative provide evidence of professionally qualified authors?

YES NO

9) Does the health site provide wording stating it is "designed to support, *not replace* PCP services (Primary Care Physicians)"?

YES NO

10) Does the health site provide a disclaimer stating that the health education content is "general information" and not "individualized patient information"?

YES NO

11) Does the health portal indicate to the visitor that his/her "confidentiality of information is secured"?

YES   NO

12) A. Does the health site provide "links" to other useful sites?

YES   NO

B. If yes, how many _____, and how many work _____ vs. "Dead Links" _____

13) Does the health portal indicate there is a formal review process (i.e., peer reviewed, editorial board)?

YES   NO

14) Provide narrative that describes the content of the site: _____
_____
_____

15) Does the health site mention the nature of audience that the site is intended for (e.g., youth vs. professional vs. elderly)?

YES   NO

16) Does the health site allow for "interaction" between the Website and user?

YES   NO

17) Cut and paste THREE "sample pages" of educational material and import into MS WORD. Indicate the average readability index: _____ grade level for these full three pages.

18) A. Is there any evidence of **"health behavior change"** theory, or the use of health/public health theories, or other theories from related fields?

YES   NO

B. If yes, indicate the theory: _____

19) Does the health site "send cookies" to your hard drive? One must standardize the number of clicks within the site. So, within the site, click to open THREE new pages/files. Indicate the number of cookies that were attached to your drive.

YES   NO

20) If yes, how many? _____ N/A

The Quality of Spanish
Health Information Websites:
An Emerging Disparity

Alberto Jose Frick Cardelle
Elaine Giron Rodriguez

East Stroudsburg University

SUMMARY. Spurred by the explosion of information technology and access to information, Internet health sites used to gather information about disease and wellness have become an accepted health education tool (Sciamanna, Clark, Houston & Diaz, 2002). There is growing evidence of concerted efforts to use the Internet to increase the access of health information to underserved populations such as Hispanics, a subpopulation with significant disparity in access to health care and health information (Hartel & Mehling, 2002). Many Hispanics are in danger of being left behind in the process, not because they reside on the wrong side of the "technology-divide," but because they reside on the wrong side of the "quality gap." Although 36% of Hispanics report having Internet access (Barreto, Ibarra, Macias & Pachon, 2000), the full advantage of the Internet requires that they have access to quality information. And while there has been significant work carried out on the reliability of health material on the Internet, only a few studies have

---

Address correspondence to: Alberto Jose Frick Cardelle, Health Services Administration Program, East Stroudsburg University, 200 Prospect Street, East Stroudsburg, PA 18301.

[Haworth co-indexing entry note]: "The Quality of Spanish Health Information Websites: An Emerging Disparity." Cardelle, Alberto Jose Frick, and Elaine Giron Rodriguez. Co-published simultaneously in *Journal of Prevention & Intervention in the Community* (The Haworth Press, Inc.) Vol. 29 No. 1/2, 2005, pp. 85-102; and: *Technology Applications in Prevention* (ed: Steven Godin) The Haworth Press, Inc., 2005, pp. 85-102. Single or multiple copies of this article are available for a fee from The Haworth Document Delivery Service [1-800-HAWORTH, 9:00 a.m. - 5:00 p.m. (EST). E-mail address: docdelivery@haworthpress.com].

looked at the quality of the health information on the Web written in Spanish (Berland et al., 2001).

In this study, 10 health themes were searched using popular search engines to generate fifty health Websites aimed at providing Spanish speakers health information. The sites were then evaluated by two raters using a 16-question assessment tool that was validated in previous research done on Internet health Websites. Summated Kappa coefficients on the reviewer ratings were found to have high inter-rater reliability ($r = .78$).

The results of this evaluation indicated that there is significant variability in the quality of health information on the Web. Furthermore, this lack of consistency in quality in health Websites is more likely to be seen in those developed and managed within Spanish-speaking countries in Latin America, the Caribbean and Europe. The article concludes that a mechanism should be developed to standardize the quality of the health information on the Internet, and to ensure the Internet as a promising vehicle through which to eliminate health disparities in Spanish populations. *[Article copies available for a fee from The Haworth Document Delivery Service: 1-800-HAWORTH. E-mail address: <docdelivery@haworthpress.com> Website: <http://www.HaworthPress. com> © 2005 by The Haworth Press, Inc. All rights reserved.]*

KEYWORDS. Internet, health literacy, health disparities, self-help, quality assurance, Hispanics

INTRODUCTION

Since the advent of the World Wide Web, health information sites continue to evolve as an important innovative resource of health information for millions of consumers. However, the continued adoption of this innovation is in jeopardy if quality assurance measures are not enacted. This article discusses how the cultural characteristics of the Hispanic population as well as the potential of the Internet as a health education tool have spurred efforts to reach Hispanics using the Internet. The article concludes by reviewing the quality assessment results of 50 Spanish health Websites and providing some general recommendations for the future of the Internet as a health education tool.

In March 2002, the Pew Internet and American Life Project estimated that 73 million Americans have used the Internet for health information, and that six million Americans go online everyday for health advice (Rainie, 2002). Consumers are increasingly using the Internet to learn more about health topics that they would be asking their primary care physicians (Diaz, Griffith, Reinert, Friedmann & Moulton, 2002). With over 100,000 health-related Web sites, the Internet is thoroughly changing the way that consumers access health information and health care (Eysenbach, 2002). Tom Ferguson, senior Research Associate at the Pew Internet and American Life Project, believes that the patients they have studied have become so capable of evaluating the health and medical information on health Websites that the term "patient" is no longer applicable and should be replaced with the term "medical end user" (Ferguson, 2002). Ferguson found that a Web user's typical one-hour search session of reputable health sites provides the user with significant health information which many primary care physicians are unacquainted (Ferguson, 2002).

A critical factor in the rise of the health sites is the multiplicity of Internet use. The use of the Internet as a communication tool in turn increases the use of the Internet as an information-gathering tool. In today's culture, families who have a member diagnosed with an illness, or in need of services from the health system, will either access the Internet or inform friends and relatives savvy with the Internet. In turn, the family and friends will not only respond with messages of support, but with specific health information they have garnered from Internet sites (Ferguson, 2002). Forty-three percent of online health searchers stated that the last time they went online they searched for materials related to their own health concerns, while 54% searched on behalf of someone else (Ferguson, 2000). The potential of the Internet to drastically change the relationship between the health care system and consumers has encouraged many organizations to view the Internet as an ideal tool to reach underserved populations such as Hispanics. Given the health disparities and the prevalence of chronic diseases faced by Hispanics, and the cultural characteristics of Hispanics, many see the Internet as an effective vehicle with which to provide Hispanics with key health information.

Hispanic Health Disparities

As the United States increasingly grows diverse, minority groups are expected to grow faster than the population as a whole. The increase among these groups is due to higher immigration and higher birth rates. By 2010, ethnic and racial minorities will constitute 32% of the total U.S. population. Within these groups, Hispanics[1] are the fastest growing minority population. Currently, approximately 35% of the total Hispanic population within the U.S. is younger than 18 years, and Hispanics have the greatest fertility rate of any ethnic group resulting in triple the growth rate of the overall U.S. population (United States Census, 2001). Hispanics currently represent 12% of the U.S. population, and by 2050 Hispanics are expected to constitute one-quarter of the United States' population (United States Census, 2000).

In addition to their population growth, Hispanics in the United States continue to have disproportionately high incidence and prevalence rates of chronic and infectious diseases. For example, the prevalence of Type 2 diabetes is two times greater in Hispanics as compared to non-Hispanic whites. Diabetes affects nearly one in four Mexican Americans (23.9%), more than one in four Puerto Ricans (26.1%), and nearly one out of six Cuban Americans (15.8%) (American Diabetes Association, 2000). Regarding infectious diseases such as HIV/AIDS, Hispanics represent 45% of the recently diagnosed AIDS cases. Of the 750,000 cumulative AIDS cases reported to CDC through June 2000, Hispanics accounted for 18% of all AIDS cases. In addition, Hispanics also account for 20% of all AIDS cases among women and 23% of the total AIDS cases among children (CDC, 2000).

Hispanics, especially Hispanic adolescents, are more likely to engage in risky sexual behaviors. Hispanics have the highest teen birth rate among the major racial/ethnic groups in the U.S. (Ventura, Martin, Curtin & Mathews, 1998). While two out of five women in the U.S. become pregnant at least once as a teen, for Hispanic women this proportion is three out of five (Day, 1996). In 1999, the birth rate for Hispanic female 15-19 year olds was 93.4 per 100,000–nearly double the national rate of 49.6 per 100,000 (Ventura, Martin, Curtin, Menacker & Hamilton, 2001). Nationally, among sexually active teen girls aged 15 to 19, 48% of Hispanic teens reported that they did not use contraception the last time they had sex, versus 32% of all sexually active teens. Also in 1995, only 29% of sexually active Hispanic males aged 15 to 19 reported using condoms consistently (100% of the time) in the previous 12 months, versus 44% of all sexually active teen males aged 15 to 19 (Moore, Driscoll & Lindberg, 1998).

Hispanics also face significant barriers to health care and health information. Health insurance is a resource that is often inaccessible to Hispanics. Hispanics are more likely to be uninsured than any other ethnic group. More than one-third of Hispanics (33.5%) are uninsured as compared with 14% of white, non-Hispanics and 20% of African Americans (Flaskerud & Kim, 1999). When compared with U.S.-born children with U.S.-born parents, immigrant children with immigrant parents were six times more likely to lack health insurance (Granados,

Puwula, Berman & Dowling, 2001). Lack of insurance becomes a major barrier for seeking health care services and for having an accessible source of health care. In fact, compared with white, non-Hispanics, Hispanics are nearly twice as likely to lack access to primary health care. This problem continues to worsen. In a study conducted by Weinick and colleagues, a review of data from three nationally representative medical expenditures surveys found that Hispanics lacking a source of primary care increased from 19.9% in 1977 to 29.5% in 1996 (Weinick, Zuvekas & Cohen 2000). Other studies have shown that Hispanic adolescents born in the U.S. are 19% more likely to use emergency rooms or public clinics as their usual source of care (Rew, 1998).

For recent immigrants and for elderly Hispanics, language is a major barrier in attaining appropriate health care services and health education (Talavera, Elder & Velasquez, 1997). Compared to all other minority groups in the United States, Hispanic adults report the fewest years of schooling (just over 10 years), and are more likely than white, non-Hispanic adults to perform in the lowest two literacy levels (Kirsch, Jungeblut, Jenkins & Kolstad, 2001). In many urban areas with high percentages of recent immigrants, more than a quarter of Hispanics report that language problems are the single greatest barrier to accessing health care. For 15% of Hispanics living in large urban areas, the barrier emerges because of a lack of Spanish-speaking physicians, and another 11% find the lack of interpreters an obstacle (Pitkin Derose & Baker, 2000). This limited English proficiency engenders lower use of health services. Hispanics with limited English may be kept from expressing their health problems, seeking preventive care, understanding doctors' instructions, and complying with treatments.

The burden of chronic and infectious diseases faced by Hispanics is compounded by disparities they face in accessing health care. These disparities include inadequate health insurance, inability to attain adequate diagnoses, lack of culturally and linguistically appropriate prevention programs, and living conditions that engender risky behaviors.

The epidemiologic profile of the U.S. Hispanic subpopulation as well as their low levels of access to primary care amplifies the attraction of using the Internet as a vehicle for increasing health information and as a tool for empowerment. While English-speaking consumers demand higher quality Internet-based health information, so too should Hispanics, who face greater barriers to traditional sources of medical care and information (Berland et al., 2001).

Internet Use Among Hispanics

Spanish-surnamed households are connecting to the Web at rapid rates. Hispanic households are purchasing computers at twice the rate of the overall population and are adopting the Internet in record numbers (*Hispanic Times Magazine*, 1999). Computer ownership in U.S. Hispanic households increased 68% over the past two years as compared with 43% in the general population. Forty-two percent of U.S. Hispanic households now have computers (Moraga, 2002). Internet penetration rates have grown each year and now stand at 30% for Hispanic households, up from 21% in 1999. We can extrapolate from these results and estimate that approximately nine million Hispanics in the U.S. are currently accessing the Internet (Barreto, Ibarra, Macias & Pachon, 2000).

Fifty percent of Hispanic users report that they access Websites that are specifically dedicated to Hispanic/Latin American issues. This study also revealed that two-thirds of Hispanic Internet users prefer using English language Websites, while 37% still prefer Spanish or bilingual Websites (Barreto, Ibarra, Macias & Pachon, 2000). According to the Tomás Rivera Policy Institute (TRPI), the outlook for future Hispanic Internet use is significant. Of Hispanics who currently do not use the Internet, a significant portion estimate that they will gain access within six months. This translates to a population that has a core group made up of established and experienced users and a growing number of new users. As with most other segments of the population, Hispanics tend to predominantly use the Internet at home (62%) compared to at work (25%) or at school (9%) (Barreto, Ibarra, Macias & Pachon, 2000). Hispanics report that research/information gathering was the number one use of the Internet followed by e-mail, reading news, business/work-related tasks, and chatting online.

Among Hispanics, there is a growing number of Internet users using the Web for gathering health information. However, while there are tens of thousands of health sites on the Internet for the English-speaking world, there are very few of any substance offered in Spanish (Bosch, 2000). Therefore this growing need for health information in Spanish and the limited existing Internet resources is a growing disparity and a challenge for health educators (Mehling, 2002). Fueled in part by the Title VI of the Civil Rights Act, organizations that receive federal funding are mandated to provide language assistance and translation of vital documents and information to individuals of limited English proficiency. With this mandate, there has been a small but growing movement among traditional health care providers and by health educators to offer Hispanics culturally competent health information through the Internet. In 2001, the U.S. Department of Health and Human Services launched the Spanish version of Healthfinder®, a Federal Website designed as a key resource for finding the best government and nonprofit health and human services information on the Internet. Also in 2001 adam.com Inc., a creator and syndicator of health information, launched DrTango.com, a provider of health- and medical-related applications and content in Spanish, and translated *Adam's Health Illustrated Encyclopedia, Surgeries and Procedures, Pregnancy Health Center*, and *Child Safety Health Center* into Spanish. In addition, medical reference services are being encouraged to supply Hispanic clients with appropriate Spanish health Websites (Mehling, 2002). Traditional health education programs such as those sponsored by the National Cancer Institute foresee using public Internet access in places such as public libraries to reach the Hispanic population with cancer prevention messages and programs (Gonzalez, 2001). And yet other programs are using the Internet to increase the cultural competency of health providers (Hilgenberg & Schlickau, 2002).

METHODS

This study identified the Spanish health Websites by searching for information on 10 health topics using four popular search engines (dogpile.com, hotbot.com, altavista.com, and google.com). The first five usable Spanish sites for each topic were accessed to be included in this evaluation study (see Table 1).

Using a previously validated assessment instrument consisting of 16 questions, two independent reviewers assessed the sampled health Websites (see Table 2) (Godin et al., 2002).

Cohen's Kappa was used to measure the degree of agreement between the two raters on questions with yes-no answers. (Cohen's Kappa measures the degree of agreement between raters on categorical assessments.) Kappa scores were calculated and summated, with the summated score divided by the number of items (see Table 3). The inter-item, inter-rater composite score was $r = .78$; this reliability coefficient suggests reasonable inter-rater agreement (Landis & Kich, 1977). The Kappa score for all the questions were $r = .6$ or above (substantial agreement) except for the item that asked reviewers to determine if the site "contained advertisements that posed a conflict of interest" (Kappa = .38 or fair agreement). The low inter-rater score with this item was most

TABLE 1. Spanish Health Websites

Sites Evaluated	
gorinka.com	dletanet.com
cancerweb.nciac.uk	unizar.es
kidshealth.org	aecc.es
gaycostarica.com	ninds.nih.gov
saludnutricion.com	sarenet.es/Parkinson
cuerpo8.es	diabetes.about.com
geocites.com	derquipilar.com
ctgrupo4.com	osteo.org/a139sp.
she-lelha.org	methodishealth.com/Spanish/womens/osteogen
tusalad.org	lungusa.org
haciendadellago.com	cdc.gov
asthme-reality.com	fwhc.org/spabort.htm
pananet.com	cidadfutura/temassalud/apendicitis
msc.es/sida	mlpediatra.mx/infantil/ulceras.htm
coscsdepeques.com	aaiba.com.arl
obesinet.roche.com	usuarias.arnet.com.ar
aids-sida.org	epilepsla.org
epilepsia-bcn.org	tuotromedico.com
methodshealth.com	elmundosalud.com
clubmedicina.com	apollocenter.com
tuotromedico.com/temas/apendicectomia.htm	delbebe.com
bulimarexia.com.ar	tupediatra.com
acidez.net	prenatal.net/embarazo.htm
adioscalvicie.com	comenzardenuevo.org
	familydoctor.org/spanish/e063.html

likely due to the fact that the question asks raters to assess the existence of a conflict of interest due to types of advertising placed on the site. Since conflict of interest is a subjective measure and difficult to operationalize given the criteria provided, reviewers were less likely to come to an agreement on this item.

Readability of the Internet Site

In order to measure the readability of the language, narrative was randomly selected from the health information text of a given educational

TABLE 2. Quality Assurance Rating Tool for Internet Health Sites

1. Is a "Name, affiliation, credentials of the author" listed on the Website?
2. Does the Website provide "References/citations" for the visitor to access should he/she wish to do further investigation or reading, or substantiate the Website material?
3. Does the health Website provide contact information and/or mail addresses for visitors to contact should he/she have further questions (check "contact us")?
4. Does the site provide any *advertisements*?
    A. If yes, do these advertisements pose potential conflicts of interest?
    B. If yes, does the Website keep advertising information *separate* from main body of health information?
5. Does the health Website cite financial support for the Website?
6. Does the health Website provide a "date of the most recent update"? Make sure it states "The site has been updated," and not have just a "date-counter."
7. Does the health Website provide evidence of professionally qualified authors?
8. Does the health Website provide wordage stating it is "designed to support, *not replace* PCP services (Primary Care Physicians)"?
9. Does the health Website provide a disclaimer stating that the health education content is "general information" and not "individualized patient information"?
10. Does the health Website indicate to the visitor's his/her "confidentiality of info is secured"?
11. A. Does the health Website provide "links" to other useful sites?
    B. If yes, how many, and how many work versus how many are "Dead Links"?
12. Does the health Website indicate there is a formal review process (i.e., peer reviewed, editorial board)?
13. Rate the "ease of determining the quality assurance"?
    5 = very difficult, 4 = difficult, 3 = neither, 2 = easy, 1 = very easy
14. Does the health Website mention the nature of audience that the site is intended for (e.g., youth vs. professional vs. elderly)?
15. Does the health Website allow for "interaction between the Website and user"?
16. Using three "sample pages" of health education material, indicate the average readability.

message/article, and pasted onto MS Word document. Using the grammar check in MS Word, a Flesch score was obtained on the readability of the text, as well as a measure on the complexity of the vocabulary and sentence structure. For Spanish documents, MS Word provides a Flesch Reading Ease Score based on a 100-point scale. The higher the score, the easier it is to understand the document. In documents for general population use, MS Word suggests a target score of approximately 60 to

TABLE 3. Kappa Scores and Their Relationship to Interrater Agreement

Kappa Score	Type of Agreement
0	Chance Agreement
0-.2	Slight Agreement
.21-.40	Fair Agreement
.41-.60	Moderate Agreement
.61-.80	Substantial Agreement
.81-.99	Almost Perfect Agreement
1.00	Perfect Agreement

(Landis & Kich, 1977)

70. In addition, MS Word gives a readability score based on rating the average number of syllables per word and words per sentence. In this scale, the higher the score the more complex the words and sentence structure.

RESULTS

The majority of the instrument's rating criteria indicate that the majority of the Spanish-language health Websites scored average to poor (see Table 4). The Websites rated the poorest with regard to the existence of a review process for accepting material for the Website. Only 3.3% of the Websites indicated that a "formal review" process existed. Seventy-two percent of the Websites did not have a confidentiality statement, while the credentials of the authors were not listed in 70% of the Websites. These three criteria are a red flag for the more educated Web surfers, and, more importantly, fail to provide the user with an adequate "trust signal."

The fact that 71% of the Websites fail to indicate that the information on the site should not serve as a substitute for a visit to a health professional is of great concern. In addition, only 32% of the Websites clearly indicated that the information on the site is not "individualized patient information." These two deficiencies are critical because they may give the user a false sense of security that he/she understands his/her condition sufficiently to self-treat or medicate. Moreover, the majority of the Websites also fail to indicate a target audience, such as the elderly or children, which can lead a user into making erroneous conclusions about their conditions.

TABLE 4. Percent of Health Websites that Have Recommended Criteria

Rating Criteria	Yes	No
Author information listed on the Website.	29.3%	70.7%
Website provides references and/or citations.	48.6%	51.4%
Site provides contact information.	90.5%	9.5%
The health Website cites its financial support.	46.4%	52.2%
The Website provides a date of the most recent update.	44.1%	55.9%
There is evidence of professionally qualified authors.	41.1%	59.9%
Website states that it is not designed to *replace* a physician's service.	28.4%	71.6%
Website states that it does not provide individualized patient information.	30.1%	68.5%
Website has confidentiality statement.	28%	72%
The Website provides "links" to other useful sites.	58.6%	41.4%
Website indicates a formal review process for the information posted.	3.3%	96.7%
Website mentions the intended target audience.	34.7%	65.3%
The Website is interactive.	62.2%	37.8%

The Websites have overall good ratings with regard to providing the user with contact information. Over 90% of the sites provide contact information, which is another vehicle by which the individual can evaluate the quality of the information. Over 60% of the Websites allow the user to interact within the Website, and 58% provide the user with links to other related health sites. Regarding links, the sites evaluated provided the user with an average of 10 useful links (Table 7). About half of the Websites provide references and citations to the health information and literature provided. Approximately half of the sites evaluated provided information on the sources of financing the site. Only about 50% of the Websites indicated the last time the site was updated. A lack of information on the last update can create uncertainty within users as they are unable to assess the timeliness of the information. Of the sites with the date of last update, 67% were updated within six months of the Webpage visit, whereas 21% had not been updated in more than 30 months (Table 6).

According to the URL, 20% of the sites identified in this study were located in other Spanish-speaking countries. Therefore, Hispanics residing in the United States will likely encounter sites providing health information written outside of the U.S. Table 5 shows the results of comparing differences between U.S.-based sites and international sites.

As measured by the raters, a greater percentage of the U.S. sites were assessed as providing higher quality information. For example, the U.S. sites

TABLE 5. Findings from the Quality Assurance Assessment of Spanish Health Websites

Rating Criteria	U.S. Based		International	
	Yes	No	Yes	No
Author information listed on the Website.	32.7%	67.3%	20%	80%
Website provides references and/or citations.	52.7%	47.3%	36.8%	63.2%
Site provides contact information.	90.7%	9.3%	90%	10%
The health Website cites its financial support.	50%	50%	38.9%	61.1%
The Website provides a date of the most recent update.	47.9%	52.1%	35%	65%
There is evidence of professionally qualified authors.	45.3%	54.7%	30%	70%
Website states that it is not designed to *replace* a physician's service.	33.3%	66.7%	15%	85%
Website states that it does not provide individualized patient information.	30.2%	69.8%	30%	70%
Website has confidentiality statement.	29.1%	70.9%	25%	75%
The Website provides "links" to other useful sites	57.7%	42.3%	61.1%	38.9%
Website indicates a formal review process for the information posted.	4.1%	95.9%	0%	100%
Website mentions the intended target audience.	32.7%	67.3%	40%	60%
The Website is interactive.	63%	37%	60%	40%

provided references and citations and evidence of professionally qualified authors 15% more than those sites managed from outside the U.S. Additionally, the U.S. sites were more likely to have statements indicating that the information on the Website should not replace a visit to a physician.

There were a few quality criteria where international sites fared better than the U.S. sites (see Table 6). International sites were more likely to indicate the target audience, or who the site was intended for. International sites were also more likely to provide the user with useful links to other health-related Websites. International sites provided the user an average of 17 links to other sites as compared to an average 8.82 links seen within the U.S.-based sites (see Table 7). The raters also found that on average, the international sites were more recently updated (Average = 8 months) as compared to the U.S. sites (Average = 13 months).

The sites showed some variability with regard to ease of use (see Table 8). Overall, over half of the sites (58.6%) were assessed by the raters as "neither easy or difficult to use," with only 7.1% rated as "very easy to use." Overall, the general pattern found was that U.S.-based sites were rated as being easier to use as compared to international sites.

TABLE 6. Number of Months Since Last Update

No. of Months	Overall	U.S.-Based Sites	International
1	37.9%	33.3%	50%
6	27.4%	24.1%	38%
12	3.4%	4.8%	0
18	6.8%	10%	0
24	3.4%	5.3%	0
More than 30	21.1%	22.5%	12%
Mean		13.57	6.3

TABLE 7. Number of Working and Useful Links to Other Health-Related Websites

No. of Sites	Overall	U.S.-Based Sites	International
1-5	45.5%	52.9%	20%
6-10	18.1%	17.7%	20%
11-15	13.7%	12.2%	20%
16-20	9.1%	5.8%	20%
21-25	8.5%	5.9%	0
More than 25	5.1%	5.5%	20%
Mean	10.4	8.82	17

TABLE 8. Ease of Use

No. of Sites	Overall	U.S.-Based Sites	International
1 very difficult to use	2.9%	2.0%	5.3%
2 difficult to use	10.0%	9.8%	10.5%
3 neither	58.6%	56.9%	63.2%
4 easy to use	21.4%	21.6%	21.1%
5 very easy to use	7.1%	9.8%	0
Mean	3.2	3.27	3

All of the Websites rated have very high readability indexes (see Table 9). There is no significant difference in readability index between the U.S. and international Websites. All of the sites were rated to have complex vocabulary with scores of 67-70 and sentences average complexity scores of 42-44. The overall Flesch readability scale of all the sites suggests a high reading level is needed by the consumers. With average Flesch scales of 7.2, the writing in these Websites requires at least a 12th grade reading level. It is important to point out that medical terms included within the educational material may have artificially inflated the readability index.

TABLE 9. Readability Scales

Criteria	Overall Mean	U.S.-Based Sites Mean	International Mean
Words per Sentence (100 = most difficult)	43.08	42.20	44.40
Vocabulary (100 = most difficult)	70.04	72.06	67.00
Flesch Scale (100 = easiest)	7.12	7.00	7.30

DISCUSSION

The Hispanic population is exploding in the United States. This demographic trend has significant implications for the health care system since it is evident that the Hispanic population has poorer health status and lower levels of access to health resources. The Internet has emerged as a cost-effective approach to providing the growing Hispanic population with the capacity to access valuable health information.

However, this study as well as others have noted that the information on health Websites are of varied quality with substantial gaps in the availability of key information (Berland et al., 2001).

The quality of the Websites evaluated for this study demonstrated gaps in quality in various areas including a tendency not to identify authors, not to provide citations and not to disclose financial support. However, the most critical deficit of the Website evaluated was their failure to provide disclaimers about how to appropriately use the information, and about the importance of seeking the services of a health professional. This is of vital importance since the target population, Hispanics, suffers from limited access and may use the information to self-treat or delay services.

Compounded with this, the study found very few health Websites geared specifically for the Hispanic population of lower education. The majority of sites had educational material with at least a 12th-grade reading level. If this high reading level represents the norm for the Internet, many of the Hispanics that witness health disparities elsewhere will witness health information that will be too difficult to read and comprehend.

Another vital factor is the role played by health Websites originating from other Spanish-speaking countries. These sites might be more attractive or more accessible to Hispanics who are recent immigrants. Unfortunately, although these sites were rated as providing more links than the U.S. sites, and slightly easier to use, they were also found to have lower quality on other important criteria.

The complexity of the information on the Internet has spurred the creation of for-profit entities that for a fee work through the deluge of information on the Internet and provide customers with a docket of information in a week (Epstein, 2003). These companies charge $150-$500 and help patients identify the most relevant information. While these entities are filling a critical niche, they are available to a small affluent segment of the population. There is an urgent need for a more universal source of quality assurance and certification. Health Websites must be encouraged to conform to certain criteria that make them truly accessible to the entire population. While the need for this certification exists for Websites of any language, health Websites targeting or aimed at underserved populations such as Hispanics need special attention. The rush to provide universal access to information should not compromise the systematic application of quality criteria and a compliance system able to enforce them. "The Internet has the potential to eliminate barriers in access to information for patients, but only if online material can be read and understood by many different types of users" (Berland et al., 2001).

The instability of the Internet is an inherent characteristic that any intervention seeking to improve quality will need to manage. Websites often disappear, change their links and even change their focus. In fact, only 30% of the sites recently assessed in this study were previously identified in a similar pilot study done the previous year (Cardelle, King & Rodriguez, 2001). With this high attrition and turnover rate, tracking Websites to provide quality assessment, credentialing and compliance enforcement will be difficult.

Unless appropriate quality assurance guidelines are implemented, the promise of the Internet as an effective health education tool for the Hispanic population will be lost. Furthermore, if the "quality gap" in the Internet continues between countries, only those more educated Hispanics will be able to benefit from the information provided thereby widening health disparities within the less educated Hispanic population.

NOTE

1. The U.S. census bureau defines persons of Hispanic origin as those who indicate that their origin is Mexican, Puerto Rican, Cuban, Central or South American, or some other Hispanic origin. Hispanics may be of any race, and may be an immigrant or someone who has been in the U.S. for generations but who has his/her roots in a Span-

ish-speaking country. Hispanics may be monolingual Spanish, monolingual English or bilingual. Since significant distinctions exist among the various Hispanic communities, there are also the important ties that transcend these differences–similarities in language, a colonial past, and, of course, a struggle against discrimination.

REFERENCES

American Diabetes Association. *Facts, Diabetes Among Hispanics*. Alexandria, VA. American Diabetes Association; 2000.

Barreto MA, Ibarra L, Macias E, Pachon H. *Latino Internet Use and Online Attitudes*. Clarement, CA. Tomás Rivera Policy Institute; 2000.

Berland GK, Elliott MN, Morales LS, Algazy JI, Kravitz RL, Broder MS, Kanouse DE, Muñoz JA, Puyol J A, Lara M, Watkins KE, Yang H, McGlynn E. Health Information on the Internet Accessibility, Quality, and Readability in English and Spanish. *JAMA*. 2001; 285: 2612-2621.

Cardelle AJ, Godin S, Rodriguez E. *Connecting Latinos: A Quality Assurance Rating System for Internet Health Portals*. American Public Health Association annual meeting. 2001; Atlanta.

Center of Disease Control and Prevention. *Semi-Annual HIV/AIDS Surveillance Report*. Atlanta. Center for Disease Control and Prevention Atlanta; 2000.

Cornelius LJ. The Degree of Usual Provider Continuity for African and Latino Americans. *J. Health Care Poor Underserved*. 1997; 8: 170-185.

Day J C. Population Projections of the United States by Age, Sex, Race, and Hispanic Origin: 1995 to 2050. *Current Population Reports*. 1996; 25-1130.

Diaz JA, Griffith RA, Reinert SE, Friedmann PD, Moulton AW. Patients' Use of the Internet for Medical Information. *J Gen Intern Med*. 2002; 17: 180-185.

Epstein RH. Shifting Through the Online Medical Jumble. *New York Times*, January 28, 2003.

Eysenbach G, Kohler C. How Do Consumers Search for and Appraise Health Information on the World Wide Web? Qualitative Study Using Focus Groups, Usability Tests, and In-depth Interviews. *BMJ*; 324: 573-577.

Ferguson T. Online Patient-Helpers and Physicians Working Together: A New Partnership for High Quality Health Care. *BMJ*; 321: 1129-1132.

Ferguson T. From Patients to End Users. *BMJ*;324: 555-556.

Fernandez Bosch, I. Hispanic Internet. *Hispanic*. 2000; 7: 22-24.

Flaskerud JH, Kim, S. Health Problems of Asian and Latino Immigrants. *Nursing Clinics of North America*. 1999; 34: 359-380.

Flores G. Culture and the Patient-Physician Relationship: Achieving Cultural Competency in Health Care. *J Pediatrics*. 2000; 136: 14-23.

Freiman MP. The Demand for Healthcare Among Racial/Ethnic Subpopulations. *Health Services Research*. 1998; 33: 867-899.

Godin S, Coke N, Daley M, Gimenez M, Miele C, Rose E, Scheffner S, Sposito J, Xu J. *Development of a Quality Assurance Rating System for Internet Disease Management Sites*. American Public Health Association annual meeting. 2000; Boston.

Gonzalez E. Cancer Education Program for Hispanics. Unpublished manuscript. Philadelphia. Fox Chase Cancer Center; 2001.

Granados G, Puwula J, Berman N, Dowling P. Health Care for Latino Children: Impact of Child and Parental Birthplace on Insurance Status Access to Health Services. *Am J Public Health*. 2001; 91: 1806-1808.

Guralnik JM, Leveille SG. Annotation: Race, Ethnicity, and Health Outcomes–Unraveling the Mediating Role of Socioeconomic Status. *Am J Public Health*. 1997; 87: 728.

Hartel LJ, Mehling R. Consumer Health Services and Collections for Hispanics: An Introduction. *Med Ref Serv Q*. 2002; 21: 35-52.

Hispanic Times Magazine. It's Here: The Latino Internet Explosion has Arrived. Op-ed. *Hispanic Times Magazine*. 1999; 5: 24.

Hilgenberg C, Schlickau J. Building Transcultural Knowledge Through Intercollegiate Collaboration. *J Transcult Nurs*. 2002;13: 241-247.

Houston T, Allison JJ. Users of Internet Health Information: Differences by Health Status. *J Med Internet Res*. 2002; 4: e7.

Kirsch IS, Jungeblut A, Jenkins L, Kolstad A. *Adult Literacy in America: A First Look at the Results of the National Adult Literacy Survey*. Washington, DC. National Center for Education Statistics; 2001.

Landis J, Kich G. The Measurement of Measurer Agreement for Categorical Data. *Biometrics*. 1977; 33: 159-174.

Moore KA, Driscoll AK & Lindberg LD. *A Statistical Portrait of Adolescent Sex, Contraception, and Childbearing*. Washington, DC. The National Campaign to Prevent Teen Pregnancy; 1998.

Moraga, F. Hispanics Are Fastest-Growing Ethnic Internet Users in Nation. *Ventura County Star*; Aug 26, 2002.

Pitkin Derose K, Baker DW. Limited English Proficiency and Latinos' Use of Physicians Services. *Medical Care Research and Review*. 2000; 57: 76-91.

Rainie L. *Health Care and the Internet Survey*. Washington, DC. Pew Charitable Trust; 2002.

Rainie L, Fox S. *Vital Decisions: How Internet Users Decide What Information to Trust When They or Their Loved Ones Are Sick*. Washington, DC. Pew Charitable Trust; 2002.

Rew L. Access to Health Care for Latinas Adolescents. *J Adolescent Health*. 1998; 23: 194-204.

Rew L, Resnick M, Beuhring T. Usual Source Patterns of Utilization, and Forgone Health Care Among Hispanic Adolescents. *J Adolescent Health*. 1999; 25: 406-412.

Sciamanna CN, Clark MA, Houston TK, Diaz JA. Unmet Needs of Primary Care Patients in Using the Internet for Health-related Activities. *J Med Internet Res*. 2002; 4: E19.

Talavera GA, Elder JP, Velasquez RJ. Latino Health Beliefs and Locus of Control: Implication for Primary Care and Public Health Practitioners. *American Journal of Preventive Medicine*. 1997; 13: 408-410.

United States Census. *Current Population Reports, Series P20-482*. Washington, DC. Population Division and Housing and Household Economic Statistics Division; 2001.

United States Census. *United States Census Bureau Report.* Washington, DC. United States Census Bureau; 2000.

Ventura SJ, Martin JA, Curtin SC, & Mathews TJ. Report of Final Natality Statistics, 1996. *Monthly Vital Statistics Report.* 1998; 46: 11s.

Ventura SJ, Martin JA, Curtin SC, Menacker F, & Hamilton BE. Births: Final Data for 1999. *National Vital Statistics Reports.* 2001; 49: 1.

Ventura SJ, Mosher WD, Curtin SC, Abma JC, & Henshaw S. Trends in Pregnancies and Pregnancy Rates by Outcome: Estimates for the United States, 1976-96. *Vital and Health Statistics.* 2000; 21: 56.

Weinick RM, Zuvekas SH, Cohen JW. Racial and Ethnic Differences in Access to and Use of Health Care Services, 1977 to 1996. *Medical Care Research & Review.* 2000; 57: 36-39.

Williams DR, Rucker TD. Understanding and Addressing Racial Disparities in Health Care. *Health Care Financing Review.* 2000; 21: 75-90.

Zambrana RE, Logie LA. Latino Child Health: Need for Inclusion in the US National Discourse. *Am J Public Health.* 2000; 90: 1827-1833.

Zuvekas SH, Weinick RM. Changes in Access to Care, 1977-1996: the Role of Health Insurance. *Health Services Research.* 1999; 34: 271-279.

A Participatory Internet Initiative in an African American Neighborhood

Yolanda Suarez-Balcazar

University of Illinois at Chicago

Leah Kinney

United Way in Chicago

Christopher M. Masi

The University of Chicago

Margaret Z. Cassey

West Suburban College of Nursing

Bashir Muhammad

Westside Health Authority

This study was conducted when Yolanda Suarez-Balcazar and Leah Kinney were at Loyola University Chicago, Center for Urban Research and Learning.

Address correspondence to: Yolanda Suarez-Balcazar, Department of Occupational Therapy (MC-811), College of Applied Health Sciences, University of Illinois at Chicago, 1919 West Taylor Street, Chicago, IL 60612.

The authors wish to thank all Citizen Leaders and all members of Every Block a Village for their involvement in this project. In addition, Claire Kohrman, Patricia Wright, Sandi Tanksley, and Harry Piotrowski assisted throughout the project. This initiative was funded, in part, by a grant from the U.S. Department of Commerce and West Suburban Health Center.

[Haworth co-indexing entry note]: "A Participatory Internet Initiative in an African American Neighborhood." Suarez-Balcazar, Yolanda et al. Co-published simultaneously in *Journal of Prevention & Intervention in the Community* (The Haworth Press, Inc.) Vol. 29, No. 1/2, 2005, pp. 103-116; and: *Technology Applications in Prevention* (ed: Steven Godin) The Haworth Press, Inc., 2005, pp. 103-116. Single or multiple copies of this article are available for a fee from The Haworth Document Delivery Service [1-800-HAWORTH, 9:00 a.m. - 5:00 p.m. (EST). E-mail address: docdelivery@haworthpress.com].

103

SUMMARY. The widespread use of technology is evident in American society, and it has become a central theme in different areas of life in the 21st century. Citizens have benefited from access to the Internet by being able to rapidly access information regarding health, housing options, employment, recreation, academics and many other areas of living. Although access to and use of the Internet has increased in all racial groups, African Americans as a group continue to have the lowest access to the Internet. This paper describes the participatory implementation and evaluation of an Internet-based intervention in an African American urban neighborhood. The project's Web page provided access to health information and health links. Forty-two Citizen Leaders (CLs), members of a grassroots group, actively participated in the different phases of the community initiative. In this paper we discuss different aspects of the planning of the intervention, its implementation, documentation of impact, maintenance and sustainability. With the introduction of technology also came lessons and challenges worth discussing. Among the challenges included recruitment of Citizen Leaders, network and hook-up problems, and Citizen Leaders' frustration in searching information on the Internet. Despite the challenges, technology became a rewarding tool for many Citizen Leaders and residents. For future directions it is critical to learn from these early efforts in order to appropriately disseminate the use of the Internet in minority communities at the neighborhood level. *[Article copies available for a fee from The Haworth Document Delivery Service: 1-800-HAWORTH. E-mail address: <docdelivery@haworthpress.com> Website: <http://www.HaworthPress.com> © 2005 by The Haworth Press, Inc. All rights reserved.]*

KEYWORDS. Internet, African Americans, technology, digital divide, Citizen Leaders

The 21st century is the century of technology. Many fields rely on technology to disseminate information, communicate with one another and transfer knowledge. In fact, the surge in use of technology is forging new definitions of *virtual communities, communications,* and *information management.* The widespread use of technology is evident in American society. Rhode and Shapiro (2000) report that over 51% of American households have in-home computers with access to the Internet. Citizens have benefited from access to the Internet by being able to rapidly access information about health, housing options, employment, recreation, academics and many other areas of living. However, not all ethnic groups are equally taking advantage of the information age; African Americans and Hispanics are falling behind and have far less access to the Internet (Spooner & Rainie, 2000).

African Americans in particular continue to be the racial group with the lowest percentage of Internet access (Rhode & Shapiro, 2000). Unfortunately, the gap between those with access and those without access to technology and the Internet is widening. This gap is often referred to as the *digital divide*. The term digital divide has been used to explain the phenomenon of differential rates of computer and Internet access based on demographic characteristics such as race and social class. Although an increase in technology training, access, and education is needed for African Americans, many minority communities lack the financial and educational resources needed to keep up with continued advances (Spooner & Rainie, 2000).

Nickelson (1998) and Sampson, Kolodinsky, and Greeno (1997) advocate Internet access for people who are geographically isolated from others or among disadvantaged communities that might not have the economic resources to pay for services. The Internet is serving as a way by which citizens can obtain support (King & Moreggi, 1998; Suler, 1999b); mental health and counseling services (Holmes, 1998; McMinn, Buchanan, Ellens, & Ryan, 1999; Stamm, 1998; Sampson, Kolodinsky, & Greeno, 1997; Suler, 1999b); obtain information about local, national and global events (Graffin & Heitkotter, 1994); obtain health information and resources (Nickelson, 1998); and facilitate communication (Preciado, 1999) among other services. Despite the potential for information overload, researchers believe that most support and health information provided through the Internet is of a positive nature. For instance, King and Moreggi (1998) found that messages that communicate support, acceptance and positive feelings were seven times more frequent than messages that communicated negative feelings in an Internet group for depressed individuals.

Access to technology has provided individuals with a powerful resource to get ahead or stay abreast in today's technological society, but at the same time, rapid developments in technology are leaving behind those who don't have access to the Internet (Rhode & Shapiro, 2000). This article describes the implementation of a community technology intervention with the goal of providing technology access and health information to an African American urban community. For the purpose of this article, the authors will use an adaptation of Linney and Wandersman's (1991) framework and Fawcett, Suarez-Balcazar, Balcazar, White, Paine, Embree, and

Blanchard's (1994) intervention research framework to report the implementation of the WebTV initiative. A WebTV is an Internet access device that can be connected to a television set. We will discuss the planning of the intervention, the implementation of the community initiative, its impact, maintenance and sustainability. We will also discuss some of the challenges encountered by the partnership team.

PARTICIPATORY DEVELOPMENT AND IMPLEMENTATION OF EVERY BLOCK A VILLAGE ONLINE

Planning Activities

Collaborative Partners. In the fall of 1998, a partnership was created with the overall goal of providing residents of an urban community with the skills and equipment necessary to access the Internet and the project's Website with mostly health information and local news. The partnership, consisting of a community-based organization called Westside Health Authority (WHA) and a community hospital called West Suburban Medical Center (WSMC), was funded by the U.S. Department of Commerce and WSMC. A local health center from the community and a local university also joined the partnership to assist with the health and participatory evaluation aspects, respectively, of the project. Partnership members embraced values and principles of community-university collaborative endeavors in which members' relationship was characterized by trust, respect, and equal participation of all members (see Suarez-Balcazar, Davis, Ferrari, Nyden, Olson, Alvarez, Molloy, & Toro, 2004; Suarez-Balcazar & Orellana-Damacela, 1999). Adhering to principles of Participatory Action Research, community partners designed the intervention and maintained control of the initiative (Balcazar, Keys, Kaplan, & Suarez-Balcazar, 1988; Jason, Keys, Suarez-Balcazar, Taylor, Davis, Durlak, & Isenberg, 2004; Selener, 1997).

WHA is a community-based organization which offers a number of community development initiatives in a working class neighborhood on Chicago's west side. WHA has been a catalyst for improving both the physical and economic condition of residents of the community through community organizing efforts. One such grassroots effort is *Every Block is a Village (EBV)*. Following from the African proverb "It Takes a Village to Raise a Child," WHA posed the question to the community, "What does it take to create a village?" The answer evolved into the EBV initiative. EBV has a membership of approximately 100 residents of the Austin community and a mission to discover and use the skills and capacities of residents to build a safe village by nurturing and supporting youth activities, building the community's infrastructure by preserving and upgrading property values, and improving and beautifying the EBV area. Once a month, 20-40 Citizen Leaders (CLs) gather at WHA for an action-planning meeting. The EBV grassroots group became the channel of the initiative called Every Block a Village Online (EVBOnline–www.ebvonline.org).

Selection of Participants. CLs, members of the EBV grassroots group, were either self-selected or were asked to participate in this initiative based upon their leadership skills and ability to connect with other residents in their neighborhood. Participants in this initiative included 42 CLs who lived in 42 different blocks in the area. All participants were African American residents. Seventy-six percent of participants were female and 24% male; 76% were between the ages of 30 and 64 years old; 12% were over 65; and 12% were between 18 and 29 years old. CLs had lived in the community for an average of 16 years, and 90% volunteered in the community (see Masi, Suarez-Balcazar, Cassey, Kinney, & Piotrowski, 2003a; Suarez-Balcazar & Kinney, 2002).

Planning Meetings and Focus Group. Representatives from WHA and WSMC met with members of EBV to discuss the planning of the WebTV initiative. EBV members discussed ways to recruit additional members and identified potential issues of community concern, such as difficulty in obtaining information about services and resources in the community, safety and health concerns, and the need to disseminate more health information to the community. In addition, members had the opportunity to talk about myths and feelings they had about technology. All of their concerns were considered in the planning of the Web page and WebTV training. Participants formed an EBVOnline research team, which met once a week for three years. The team included representatives from all partners including a doctor from the hospital, a nurse with expertise in public health who also served as the Webmaster, the technology coordinator for WHA, staff from WHA, members of the community, members of EBV, and community researchers.

Implementation of the Every Block a Village Online Initiative

CLs who volunteered for the EVBOnline project completed an initial 30-minute interview, conducted by the researchers and two trained community residents. The interview included structured questions regarding constructs such as sense of community, community empowerment, use and attitudes toward technology and basic demographic questions. The same interview was conducted 12 months later. After the interview, each CL received a 90-minute WebTV training session which included: (a) basic use of WebTV, (b) how to send emails to others, and (c) how to access the project's Web page, health links and the project's 24-hour Ask-a-Doc service staffed by WSMC. At the end of training, the technology coordinator scheduled an appointment with the CL to install the WebTV, provide the CL with a printer, paper and information on how to obtain troubleshooting services and technical support as needed. The equipment was provided to CLs at no cost. CLs were encouraged to meet regularly with their neighbors to talk about the availability of additional WebTVs at public sites such as WHA, the recreation center, and a nearby high school. They were also encouraged to print information of relevance to the community (e.g., meetings, announcements, services) and disseminate it to their neighbors, relatives and friends. Initially, the project team encouraged members to let other neighbors into their homes to use WebTV; however, CLs decided that was not desirable because of safety reasons. Instead, CLs could let others on their block know about the availability of units at public sites or offer to do an Internet search for them.

Participatory Aspects of the Initiative. To shape the WebTV intervention to meet the needs of the community we maintain a system of ongoing involvement and feedback from residents and leaders. Team members designed an EBVO Web page with EBV CLs' feedback and their active involvement. For instance, CLs selected the logo for EBVO. Because of the project's heavy emphasis on health and safety, links to information about community services and health information were added. Furthermore, the Web page also became a message board for community announcements on upcoming meetings, events and services. The Web page changed as feedback from members continued. During Black History Month, CLs requested to have a vast set of resources and links to African American culture so the children in the community could learn and do their homework. In late summer, the Web page contained information about medical forms, vaccinations sites, and how to get kids ready for school.

In order to maintain ongoing contact with all CLs (beyond the one who participated in the weekly team meetings), the team designed a 5-minute phone interview. This interview was conducted every three to four weeks and asked CLs to report how often they had used WebTV, topics they searched for, successful attempts at obtaining information, problems they might be having and sites and links they would like to see on the project's Web page. Every time the CLs reported trouble with the unit, the technology coordinator and two trained teenagers from the community provided troubleshooting assistance. Furthermore, during the last year of the project, a CL and WHA staff received ongoing training on how to maintain the project's Web page.

Participatory Evaluation

Team members embraced a participatory and empowerment approach to documenting impact of the initiative (see Masi et al., 2003a; Masi et al., 2003b; Suarez-Balcazar, Orellana-Damacela, Portillo, Sharma, & Lanum, 2003; Suarez-Balcazar & Harper, 2003). Team members developed a project's logic model and identified several methodologies and sources of data to document process and intermediate outcome indicators. Process documentation took place through ongoing 5-minute phone interviews and collection of Web stories (see Suarez-Balcazar & Kinney, 2002). Two community residents received training on how to conduct these phone interviews, and the information and feedback collected was used at weekly meetings and incorporated into the Web page to meet the needs of community residents. Furthermore, we analyzed the content of e-mails that made it to the listserv and interviewed CLs about their perspectives on the project. For intermediate outcomes, the team used a nonequivalent comparison group designed to examine pre- and post-ratings on sense of community, sense of empowerment and attitudes toward technology (Masi et al., 2003a; Masi et al., 2003b; Suarez-Balcazar, 2003). These various documentation methods have lead the research team to view the impact of the intervention in many different ways. For the purpose of this paper, we will be describing some of the uses of WebTV, e-mails, and CL perspectives on the project including a pre- and post-intervention structured interview (Masi, Suarez-Balcazar, Cassey, Kinney, & Piotrowski, 2003).

Citizen Leaders' Use of WebTV. Through the ongoing follow-up phone interviews team members gathered information on the uses of WebTV, successful and unsuccessful attempts at obtaining information, uses of the information, and sharing of information (see Masi et al., 2003a). Overall, CLs used WebTV an average of three times a week. In addition, relatives, friends and neighbors of CLs also used WebTV about once a week. From a total of 450 Web stories (successful gathering of information) reported, 43% of the stories were about information gathered for the CL; 29% of the stories were about relatives obtaining and using the information; 15% of the stories alluded to neighbors obtaining and using the information; and 13% of the stories were about the community benefiting from the information (e.g., Citizen Leader passing information, obtained through the Web page, at a block meeting about street lights) (Suarez-Balcazar & Kinney, 2002). Fourteen percent of the stories referred to health-related information (e.g., checking the side effects of a prescription, a pregnant Citizen Leader obtaining information about healthy eating, obtaining information on how to reduce asthma triggers). In addition, the team also content-analyzed 577 e-mails that were sent to the entire CL listserv. Table 1 illustrates the type of e-mails according to their purpose. The e-mail listserv primarily facilitated the dissemination of information about community events and resources in the community. Furthermore, members used the WebTV to provide spiritual support through daily religious messages and citations from the Bible. It is important to note that this is a very spiritual community. All EBV meetings began and ended with an uplifting prayer.

During CL post-intervention assessments, researchers recorded comments on the personal impact the unit had in their lives. Table 2 provides examples of the personal comments recorded from Citizen Leaders. Although some CLs thought it was hard to search and the machines were slow in connecting, Citizen Leaders were generally very satisfied with their new skills and equipment. Interestingly, CLs began to report the speed of connection as an issue after they got better at using WebTV; at first, it took time to learn the new skills so connecting didn't seem an issue. One CL who home-schooled her three children reported that she used WebTV as a teaching tool and had been successful at connecting to educational links to teach her kids.

Residents' Use of WebTV. Seven public sites were provided with the WebTV equipment and staff training. A phone interview was con-

TABLE 1. Percent of E-Mail Type

Type of E-Mail	
Information (community services and resources, announcements about events and citizen rights)	42%
*Spiritual	29%
Encouragement	12%
Request for participation	8%
Reminder about community meeting	6%
Report of community action	3%

*Note: Despite the fact that 29% of e-mails exchanged contained *only* spiritual messages, about 80% of all other e-mails included a cite or story from the Bible at the end of the message.

TABLE 2. Sample of Citizen Leaders' Personal Views on the Impact of WebTV on Their Lives

- "I have been able to maintain regular communication with family, friends, and neighbors"
- "As a Citizen Leader using WebTV I have been able to help my community much better"
- "WebTV has opened awareness about new information, has given me easy access to information"
- "I feel tremendous pride in my new skill, I have access to something I did not have before, and thought it was not for me"
- "At the beginning of the project using WebTV was too overwhelming, now I feel very comfortable using it"
- "I never used e-mail before, now I know what it is, I used it a lot and love it"
- "My health is much better now that I use WebTV for health information and resources"
- "It helped empower me, it changed my life because I have a new way of gaining access to information and resources"
- "It has allowed me help others better by passing out information and communicating"
- "I became more knowledgeable, more educated, came in contact with things I never thought about"
- "I feel empowered because I have a sense of what is happening in my community and the world"
- "It has given me more easy and inexpensive (Ask a Doc) access to health information, resources and advice"

ducted with a staff member of the site between three to six months after placement of the unit to assess the frequency of WebTV use in these public sites. These sites included recreation centers, after-school programs, WHA and a local high school. Before the placement of WebTVs, residents of this community had minimal public access to the Internet. Sites were provided with staff training, the WebTV unit, a printer and troubleshooting by the technology coordinator of the center. In all, five out of the seven sites reported actively using their WebTV. The most frequent users were children and teenagers, most commonly for entertainment purposes, to do homework, and look for employment information. On average, 25 kids used WebTV daily at each of the five public sites. In addition, staff at three of the sites reported parents also coming to use the unit. The following comments were reported from staff: "Kids love the unit," "The kids often fight for it so we had to set limits and the priority is homework," "The WebTV is very popular with the kids," "A few of the kids brought their parents, to try it out" and "Many of our kids did not know what the Internet was and now they love it."

Intervention Maintenance and Sustainability

During the final year of the three-year project, the team's Webmaster transferred the control of the Web page to the community with the assistance of the technology coordinator and staff from WHA. In addition, the community-based organization (WHA) received funding for a local technology center, which was facilitated by this initiative. Furthermore, WHA staff encouraged many CLs to invest in personal computers. The technology center is currently run by the Technology Coordinator for WHA, CLs who are members of EBV, and community residents, in particular community youth. Currently, many of the technology center users are teenagers, who have also become instructors to adults or younger kids. The center has about 15 personal computers with access to the Internet.

CHALLENGES AND LESSONS LEARNED

The introduction of technology is not necessarily smooth and easy. During the planning stage, it was difficult to recruit new CLs. We had planned to train at least 30 or so CLs during the first year and it took over 2 years to have all 42 trained. This occurred in part because of delays in securing CLs who wanted to be trained and delays in obtaining the equipment.

With the benefits of technology come various technical failures such as network and connection problems that hindered learning progress and triggered frustration among CLs. Although the team provided ongoing monitoring and support, there were numerous connection delays and problems. Additionally, some CLs noticed a slight increase in their local phone expenses due to calling into the network. Lastly, as CLs began to share information with their community, they raised concerns about the safety of allowing neighbors into their homes or walking around the streets distributing information; therefore, CLs and WHA staff encouraged residents to use public sites and the new technology center.

FUTURE DIRECTIONS

For urban communities to take advantage of information technology, technology needs to be introduced at the individual and community levels and tailored to the needs of the community. In this study, WebTVs were introduced into the homes of CLs and public sites in collaboration with a community organization and its grassroots group. African Americans and other minorities can benefit by having this type of supportive environment that will ultimately allow them to take advantage of the benefits provided by the use of the Internet, such as access to information and rapid communication (Rhode & Shapiro, 2000). With this study, we realized that CLs began using their WebTV units as a tool for helping themselves and engaged in community action using technology as a tool to promote community change (see Suarez-Balcazar & Kinney, 2002). As stated by Francisco, Fawcett, Schultz, Berkowitz, Wolff, and Nagy (2001), technology can serve as a tool for enhancing capacity. The participatory approach taken in the development and implementation of the intervention facilitated the dissemination of information and skills building in the community. Future implementations of technology innovations in urban communities need to include an ongoing support system providing troubleshooting and opportunities for residents to share their stories and tips. Rhode and Shapiro (2000) assert the importance of providing troubleshooting and support in the learning process while acquiring technology-related skills.

Given the challenges experienced by residents in connecting and other technical problems, we realized that although the WebTV is a good place to begin and perhaps less intimidating initially than a personal computer, a personal computer (PC) might present fewer technical and logistic difficulties. In addition, we observed a learning curve. Most CLs took a few months to feel comfortable using the WebTV before they started using it regularly. However, as their competence with WebTV grew, CLs began to report problems and frustration with the units. Based on this experience, we believe that beginning with PCs and making them more accessible to low-income communities might be best rather than using WebTV units.

An important observation from this project was the openness to learning and ease with which the community's youth learned Internet-related skills. Youth from the community played a very critical role in assisting adults by providing troubleshooting and one-on-one support. In fact, in many of the Citizen Leaders' homes where there was a young child or teenager (9 years old and up), the TV unit had a lot of use, and adults reported great satisfaction in seeing the kids use the unit. As a Citizen Leader said, "I prefer to see my grandson using the unit than out on the streets looking for trouble." Future technological innovations need to focus on making the Internet available to all children and youth. They can assist in the training of the adults. Perhaps more support centers and training needs to be available at the individual and community level.

To many of the project's CLs the WebTV became a powerful resource to access information on a variety of topics including health, entertainment, housing, employment and other important areas of daily life. Future directions need to consider how to make technology even more economically available to people of scarce resources. Despite having access to PCs and WebTVs in public sites such as recreation centers, residents preferred to have technology at home. We all can associate with the comfort of having easy access to the Internet. Through this project, 42 WebTVs were distributed among residents, which resulted in about one unit per block with the initial idea of having residents visit each other's homes and share the unit with people on their block rejected by residents because of safety concerns. Although researchers (Nickelson, 1998; Sampson, Kolodinsky, & Greeno, 1997) have advocated for Internet access for people who are geographically isolated, we advocate for Internet access for urban minorities who are isolated because of poverty. Residents living in urban areas of high crime and inadequate transportation services might also feel isolated from the rest of the urban life. Having home access to the Internet with a community Web page provides residents with information about local news, events, information about resources and services. Local communities need to explore ways to make such a powerful tool economically feasible to all its residents not just to those who can afford technology.

At the end of the project, the team discussed what to do with the units and how to help members obtain PCs to continue developing their new skills. In future projects, we suggest using PCs instead of WebTVs and providing ongoing support during the learning curve. The technology center facilitated this transfer, but motivation to keep using technology appeared to be driven by satisfaction of knowing that one can find something useful and rewarding. Technology became a rewarding tool for some but was difficult for others who decided not to keep up with their newly acquired skills. Furthermore, some residents were unable to keep the WebTV units once the project ended because of the monthly fees (during the three-year duration of the project the unit and monthly fees were covered by the project). Cost is definitely an issue in making technology available to low-income communities. Many families in low-income communities see technology as a luxury they can't afford.

This study is one of the first attempts at examining the introduction of technology in a low-income African American community at the neighborhood level. By learning from these early efforts, we might be able to better disseminate the use of the Internet in low-income communities. Overall, future efforts of this kind need to examine ways to make technology units (WebTVs, PCs with access to the Internet) not only economically feasible but its monthly maintenance reasonable for families with limited resources.

REFERENCES

Balcazar, F., Keys, C. B., Kaplan, D. L., & Suarez-Balcazar, Y. (1988). Participatory action research and people with disabilities. *Canadian Journal of Rehabilitation. 12*, 105-112.

Fawcett, S. B., Suarez-Balcazar, Y., Balcazar, F., White, G., Paine, A., Embree, M. G., & Blanchard, K. A. (1994). Intervention research in communities: Methods and exemplars. In J. Rothman & E. J. Thomas (Eds.), *Intervention research: Creating effective methods for professional practice.* Chicago: University of Chicago Press.

Francisco, V. T., Fawcett, S. B., Schultz, J. A., Berkowitz, B., Wolff, T. J., & Nagy, G. (2001). Using Internet-based resources to build community capacity: The community tool box [http://ctb.ujans.edu/]. *American Journal of Community Psychology, 29*, 293-300.

Graffin, A., & Heitkotter, G. (1994). Guide to the Internet: A round trip through global networks, life in cyberspace, and everything. Retrieved 1999, from http://www. eff.org/papers/eegtti/eeg-toc.html#SEC45

Holmes, L. G. (1998). Delivering mental health services online: Current issues, *CyberPsychology and Behavior, 1*, 1, 19-24.

Jason, L. A., Keys, C. B., Suarez-Balcazar, Y., Taylor, R. R., Davis, M., Durlak, J., & Isenberg, D. (Eds.) (2004). Participatory community research: Theories and methods in action. Washington, DC: American Psychological Association.

King, S. A., & Moreggi, D. (1998). Internet therapy and self help groups–the pros and cons. In J. Gackenbach (Ed.), *Psychology and the Internet: Intrapersonal, interpersonal and transpersonal implications* (pp. 77-109). San Diego, CA: Academic Press.

Linney, J. A., & Wandersman, A. (1991). Prevention plus 111: Assessing alcohol and other drug prevention programs at the school and community level: A four-step guide to useful program assessment. Rockville, MD: U.S. Department of Health and Human Services, Office for Substance Abuse Prevention.

Masi, C. M., Suarez-Balcazar, Y., Cassey, M. Z., Kinney, L., & Piotrowski, Z. H. (2003a). Internet access and empowerment: A community-based health initiative. *Journal of General and Internal Medicine, 18*, 1-6.

Masi, C. M., Suarez-Balcazar, Y., Cassey, M. Z., Kinney, L., & Piotrowski, Z. H. (2003b). Internet access and empowerment. *Journal of General and Internal Medicine, 18(SI)*, 181.

McMinn, M. R., Buchanan, T., Ellens, B. N., & Ryan, M. K. (1999). Technology, professional practice and ethics: Survey findings and implications. *Professional Psychology: Research and Practice, 30*, 165-172.

Nickelson, D. W. (1998). Telehealth and the evolving health care system: Strategic opportunities for professional psychology. *Professional Psychology: Research and Practice, 29*, 527-535.

Preciado, J. (1999). Applicaciones de Internet a la psicologia de la salud (1999). *Suma Psicologica, 6*, 241-255.

Rhode, G. L., & Shapiro, R. J. (2000). Falling through the net: Toward digital inclusion. A report on Americans' access to technology tools. Washington, DC: The Secretary of Commerce.

Sampson, J., Kolodinsky, R. W., & Greeno, B. P. (1997). Counseling on the information highway: Future possibilities and potential problems. *Journal of Counseling and Development, 75*, 203-211.

Selener, D. (1997). *Participatory action research and social change*. Ithaca, NY: Cornell Participatory Action Research Network.

Spooner, T., & Rainie, L. (2000). African-Americans and the Internet. Pew Internet & American life project. Washington, DC: U.S. Department of Commerce.

Stamm, H. B. (1998). Clinical applications of telehealth in mental health care. *Professional Psychology: Research and Practice, 29*, 536-542.

Suarez-Balcazar, Y. (June 2003). Empowerment and participatory evaluation of community interventions: Implications for community occupational therapy. Paper presented at the American Occupational Therapy Association. Washington, DC.

Suarez-Balcazar, Y., Davis, M., Ferrari, J., Nyden, P., Olson, B., Alvarez, J., Molloy, P., & Toro, P. (2004). University-community partnerships: A framework and an exemplar. In L. Jason, C. B. Keys, Y. Suarez-Balcazar, R. R. Taylor, M. Davis, J. Durlak, & D. Isenberg (2004) Eds. *Participatory community-research: Theory and methods in action*. Washington, DC: American Psychological Association.

Suarez-Balcazar, Y., & Harper, G. (Eds.) (2003). Community-based approaches to empowerment and participatory evaluation. *Journal of Prevention & Intervention in the Community, 26*(2), 5-20.

Suarez-Balcazar, Y., & Kinney, L. (2002). Technology as a tool for facilitating community change. *The Community Psychologist, 35*, 25-27.

Suarez-Balcazar, Y., & Orellana-Damacela, L. (1999). A university-community partnership for empowerment evaluation with a community housing organization. *Journal of Clinical and Applied Sociology*, (1), 115-132.

Suarez-Balcazar, Y., Orellana-Damacela, L., Portillo, N., Sharma, A., & Lanum, M. (2003). Implementing an outcomes model in the participatory evaluation of community initiatives. *Journal of Prevention and Intervention in the Community, 26*(2), 5-20.

Suler, J. (1999b). Unique groups in cyberspace. Available: http://www.rider.edu/users/suler/psycyber/overview.html

Alcohol Abuse Prevention Among High-Risk Youth: Computer-Based Intervention

Steven P. Schinke
Traci M. Schwinn
Alfred J. Ozanian

Columbia University

SUMMARY. This study examined the feasibility of a CD-ROM intervention to prevent alcohol abuse among high-risk youths. Youths from 41 community-based agencies in greater New York City participated in a randomized trial of a skills-based interactive CD-ROM. Outcome data were collected on 489 early adolescents in these agencies before and after a randomized subset of youths interacted with a 10-session alcohol abuse prevention program on CD-ROM. Compared to control participants, youths in the intervention arm had a positive increase in perceived

Address correspondence to: Steven Schinke, School of Social Work, Columbia University, New York, NY 10025 (E-mail: Schinke@columbia.edu).

The authors extend their sincere thanks to United Neighborhood Houses, Police Athletic League, and the numerous other organizations throughout greater New York City, New Jersey, and Delaware without whose handsome support this research would not have been possible.

This research was supported in full by a generous grant from the National Institute on Alcoholism and Alcohol Abuse, AA11924.

[Haworth co-indexing entry note]: "Alcohol Abuse Prevention Among High-Risk Youth: Computer- Based Intervention." Schinke, Steven P., Traci M, Schwinn, and Alfred J. Ozanian. Co-published simultaneously in *Journal of Prevention & Intervention in the Community* (The Haworth Press, Inc.) Vol. 29, No. 1/2, 2005, pp. 117-130; and: *Technology Applications in Prevention* (ed: Steven Godin) The Haworth Press, Inc., 2005, pp. 117-130. Single or multiple copies of this article are available for a fee from The Haworth Document Delivery Service [1-800-HAWORTH, 9:00 a.m. - 5:00 p.m. (EST). E-mail address: docdelivery@haworthpress.com].

http://www.haworthpress.com/web/JPIC
Digital Object Identifier: 10.1300/J005v29n01_08

harm of alcohol use and increased assertiveness skills. At posttest, drinking rates for control and intervention participants were equal and unchanged from pretest. These findings suggest that CD-ROM technology offers a new and promising medium for engaging high-risk youth in an alcohol abuse prevention program. Study implications and future applications of the present approach are discussed. *[Article copies available for a fee from The Haworth Document Delivery Service: 1-800-HAWORTH. E-mail address: <docdelivery@haworthpress.com> Website: <http://www.HaworthPress. com> © 2005 by The Haworth Press, Inc. All rights reserved.]*

KEYWORDS. Alcohol abuse, CD-ROM, prevention, youth, computer, skill- building

Nearly one half of all U.S. youths have tried alcohol before ninth grade, and by tenth grade 50% have been drunk at least once (Centers for Disease Control and Prevention, 2000; Johnston, O'Malley, & Bachman, 2002). Expectedly, youthful drinking often antecedes adult drinking. More than 40% of individuals who start drinking before age 13 years will abuse alcohol or develop alcohol dependence as adults (Grant & Dawson, 1997). In a survey of 18- to 24-year-old current drinkers who failed to complete high school, nearly 60% had drunk alcohol before age 16 years (National Institute on Alcohol Abuse and Alcoholism, 1998). Clearly, the time to prevent alcohol abuse is before young people enter the teen years.

Prevention programs aimed at alcohol and other substance use have proven their worth (Botvin & Kantor, 2000; Scheier, Botvin, & Griffin, 2001; Schinke, Gordon, & Weston, 1990). Before they are widely disseminated and accessible, however, prevention programs must address a number of challenges. Chief among these challenges is finding a way to attract and sustain youths' attention. These engaging prevention programs must be replicable and easily disseminated, and they must lend themselves to high protocol fidelity to move from science to practice. In fact, well-implemented programs are associated with commensurately positive results (Botvin, Baker, Dusenbury, Botvin, & Diaz, 1995). Cost-containment is vital before prevention will be embraced by budget-minded education and non-profit sectors. Fortunately, many, if not all, of these obstacles to effective prevention programming may be addressed through new technologies.

Prevention and New Technologies

The marriage of prevention science and new technologies offers considerable promise. Prevention aims to deter problem behavior before it starts and, failing that, to delay the age of onset of behavior problems. With respect to youths and alcohol consumption, if drinking is delayed until age 21 years, the risk of serious alcohol problems decreases by 70% (Grant & Dawson, 1997). For prevention programs to work, they must establish and sustain connections with youth recipients. The appropriate use of new technologies is essential to making that connection.

Reviews of prevention programs for youths increasingly recognize interactive computer technology as a potential avenue for health education and intervention. Children and teenagers use computers and the Internet more than any other age group. Of those aged 5 to 17 years, 90% use computers; 75% of teenagers surf the Internet (U.S. Department of Commerce, 2002). These trends notwithstanding, investigators have only begun to experiment with technological delivery modes for prevention programming. Nearly all science-based adolescent drug abuse and other prevention programs are delivered via small group format, despite the myriad advantages to computer-based interventions (Rotheram-Borus, 2000).

CD-ROM and the Internet are the two prevailing modes for computer-based interventions. Both technologies have their advantages. The Internet can be accessed from the home, school, or such community agencies as libraries and youth service organizations. But dial-up modems, which are used by 80% of Internet users, are slow. Highly innovative interactive programs need broadband service to run optimally. Though the Internet holds greater potential, the current standard for delivering fast-paced, interactive prevention programming is CD-ROM.

CD-ROM

Youths who receive prevention programs via CD-ROM can access and navigate through topic modules at their own pace. Interactively presented content is stimulating and varied and permits skills demonstrations and guided rehearsal. Young people enjoy unique character designs and animations, complex graphics, and judiciously placed text. The branching technology available to CD-ROM programming allows for the development of multiple story lines that play according to the choices youths make. Youths benefit by interacting with tailored sessions based on their current skill level. Further, researchers cognizant of their target population can incorporate developmentally and culturally tailored audio, animation, graphics, and video into the CD-ROM.

Protocol fidelity, portability, ease of use, and data storage associated with CD-ROM technology can benefit research design and dissemination capabilities. CD-ROM allows investigators to distribute prevention programs, knowing that youths will receive the evaluated intervention. More than 10 hours of interactive content can be stored on one portable disk and delivered to anyone with access to a computer and CD-ROM drive.

Cost also favors CD-ROM. At present, a science-based, adult-led prevention program, including the necessary training and materials, costs between $500 and $900 for a classroom of 30 students. CD-ROMs greatly reduce the need for program materials and staff training; they can reach each child in a class of 30 students for a total cost of less than $60.00.

The Digital Divide

No discussion of Internet usage and computer accessibility can neglect the "digital divide." This refers to the gap between people and communities who can make effective use of new information technology and those who cannot (Digital Divide Network, 2002). Debate as to whether the "divide" is shrinking or expanding continues. In 1998, 37% of homes in the United States were equipped with computers. By 2001, that number had increased to 57%. Over those same 4 years, Internet use increased from 19% to 51% (U.S. Department of Commerce, 2002). Demographic statistics, however, reveal ethnic-racial gaps in computer ownership and Internet use.

By the end of 2001, Asian and White Americans' computer use was roughly 70%, whereas African-Americans' and Latinos' use was 56% and 49%, respectively (U.S. Department of Commerce, 2002). The digital divide is also apparent in Internet use. About 30% fewer African-Americans and Latinos are online compared to Asian and White Americans.

Minority youths with the least access to computers and the Internet are at greatest risk for substance abuse. Compared to Whites, Blacks have higher substance-related mortality and morbidity (National Cancer Institute, 1991). A higher percentage of Latino youths, compared to Whites and Blacks, have tried alcohol before they are 13 years old (Centers for Disease Control and Prevention, 2001). Despite the logic of directing prevention efforts at minority children, gaps remain in the science of preventing alcohol and other substance abuse among African-American, Latino, economically disadvantaged, and other high-risk youths. The study described in this article aimed to bridge some of those gaps. In so doing, the study examined the feasibility and preliminary effectiveness of an interactive CD-ROM designed to prevent alcohol abuse among high-risk youths.

METHODS

Setting and Participants

Study participants were 489 youths from greater New York City, and parts of New Jersey and Delaware. Youths were recruited from 43 afterschool agencies that serve economically disadvantaged children and adolescents. These sites were primarily afterschool drop-in centers, clubs, neighborhood centers, and other youth organizations. Based on Census data from 2000 and the zip codes in which the agencies are located, family household incomes were at or below the Federal poverty line of $17,050 for a family of five (U.S. Department of Health and Human Services, 2000).

Study participants assented to research involvement and their parents or legal guardians provided informed consent. Though all participants were English speaking, consent forms were made available in Spanish for parents who were not comfortable with English. The Institutional Review Board at Columbia University approved consent procedures.

At baseline 51.4% of the sample was female and the median age was 10.84 years. Most of the participants were from ethnic-racial minority groups: 54% were African-American, 30% were Hispanic, 11% were White, and 5% were from other ethnic-racial groups.

Design

Prior to pretesting, participants were randomly assigned to one of three arms: control, CD-ROM intervention, and parent-enhanced CD-ROM intervention. Eleven sites (youth $n = 160$) were assigned to the control arm and 26 sites (youth $n = 329$) were assigned to the intervention arms. Participants in the control arm completed pretest and posttest measurements only. Participants in both intervention arms completed pretest measurements, received the CD-ROM intervention, and were posttested.

Measures

On forms kept separate from other measures, informed and consenting youths reported various demographic and tracking information. Assertion skills were measured by asking youths to define the word *assertiveness* and answer questions about their ability to intercede if their friends were about to get into trouble and their ability to stop socializing with friends who could get them into trouble. This skill was measured by adapting the short form of the Children's Action Tendency Scale (Deluty, 1979, 1984). Youths' ability to perceive harm was measured on a 5-point Likert scale by asking "How often do people hurt themselves when they drink alcohol?"

Included in the schedule were questions related to self-efficacy, problem solving, educational attainment, peer interactions, and family rules related to alcohol and substance use. Peer substance use associations were measured by asking participants how many of their five closest friends drink alcohol; have ever been drunk; smoke marijuana; smoke cigarettes; sniff inhalants; or use crank, heroin, ecstasy, or any other drug. Alcohol and other substance use were self-reported.

Intervention Content

Youths in the intervention arm received the interactive CD-ROM prevention program Thinking Not Drinking: A SODAS City Adventure. Thinking Not Drinking is a skills-based program that consists of ten, 45-minute sessions. Grounded in the frameworks of social cognitive theory, problem-behavior theory, peer-cluster theory, and family-networks theory, the sessions cover goal setting, coping, media literacy, peer pressure, and assertiveness training, as well as such preventive strategies as norm correcting, decision making, and effective communication. The CD-ROM emphasizes prevention strategies thematically through a specific problem-solving sequence.

The problem-solving approach, which provides a context for learning and applying alcohol abuse prevention content, is central to other substance abuse prevention programs (Botvin, Baker, Dusenbury, Tortu, & Botvin, 1990; Botvin, Epstein, Baker, Diaz, & Ifill-Williams, 1997; Hawkins, Catalano, Kosterman, Abbott, & Hill, 1999; Schinke, Botvin, & Orlandi, 1991). The problem-solving approach also lends itself to relatively straightforward programming, provides engaging interactive material, and equips youths with a practical skill set to understand, integrate, and apply all other elements of the alcohol abuse prevention program.

Each session in the CD-ROM begins with skill-specific objectives youths must meet to advance to the next session. Navigating through an edgy urban landscape, youths encounter simulated yet realistic obstacles and distractions depicted by animated characters mimicking the age, gender, and demographic background of the target adolescents. To successfully maneuver through each session, youths must employ specific problem-solving skills. A principal character, acting as the youths' conscience, guides youths through the core problem-solving sequence of *Stop, Options, Decide, Act*, and *Self-praise*.

In the *Stop* step, youths learn to pause and define problems and to identify their responsibility in solving problems related to alcohol abuse use and other personal issues. In the second step, *Options,* youths interact with a process for learning how to generate, consider, and evaluate alternative solutions to problems. For the *Decide* step, youths choose what they consider the best solution from the generated list of alternatives by assessing each option on its costs and benefits.

In *Act*, the fourth step, youths are provided the opportunity to witness the consequences of their decision, whether or not the choice is correct. If youths pick the appropriate choice, they see the positive results of their decision making. If they select an incorrect option, they are rerouted to the original list of options, but only after they have witnessed the negative consequences of the poor decision. Youths are then asked to *Decide* and *Act* again, until the correct option is chosen and the positive consequence experienced.

In the *Self-praise* step, youths see how to reward themselves for engaging in the problem-solving sequence, regardless of the outcome of the options they selected. Since youths cannot control the way others react to their problem-solving responses in everyday situations, the self-praise step provides a predictable reward that youths can give to themselves when they correctly use problem-solving techniques–regardless of the consequences.

Procedure

Most youths completed the 10-session intervention at the collaborating afterschool agency from which they were recruited. During the course of delivery intervention, some study participants moved away from or stopped attending their afterschool program. In these instances, youths completed the intervention in the research offices or on laptop computers in their homes. Youths with adequate home computers were provided copies of the game. Each intervention session took approximately 45 minutes to complete and was intended to be completed weekly.

Columbia University research assistants collected pretest data on all 489 participants at collaborating sites. At posttest, the majority of data were collected via telephone because many youths had stopped attending their sites and others had moved beyond the study area. To protect participants' privacy, the survey delivery plan precluded family members' interpreting youths' responses. Participants received a mailer containing a survey answer booklet in advance of the telephone survey. During the posttest telephone survey, data collectors read each survey item and participants responded with the letter that represented their answer.

Data Analysis and Results

Quantitative. Outcome data were coded, cleaned, entered and analyzed according to measurement protocol for each schedule. Data analyses proceeded with SPSS for Windows.™ Table 1 shows no differences between intervention and control arms on participants' age, gender, or school grades. Family composition and race differed between the two groups. Divorced or separated households accounted for 46.3% of intervention families; only 35% of participants in the control arm were in divorced or separated families. Ethnic-racial background also was not evenly distributed between the two groups.

Gain score analyses were employed for outcome tests. These scores were derived arithmetically by subtracting participants' pretest scores from their posttest scores on the same items. By analyzing gain scores with two-sample, independent *t* tests, the significance of between-arm differences in participants' outcome scores from the pretest measurement occasion to the posttest measurement occasion was determined.

Figure 1 shows that youths assigned to the intervention arm scored more positively on assertion skills and perceived harm of alcohol than participants assigned to the control arm. At pretest, intervention and control participants scored 1.15 on a 2-point scale for assertion skills, where 1 = *wrong definition of assertion* and 2 = *correct definition*. At posttest, control participants were unchanged, and intervention participants increased to 1.36, $t(472) = 4.01$, $p < .0005$ (two-tailed).

As seen in Figure 1, participant scores at pretest did not differ significantly (Intervention = 4.20, Control = 4.24) when asked to rate their perceived harm of alcohol on a 5-point scale, with 1 = *never harmful* and 5 = *always harmful*. At posttest, intervention participants scored higher

TABLE 1. Demographic Characteristics of Study Population

	CD and Parent Group ($n = 329$) %	Control ($n = 160$) %	df	χ^2	p
Age (in years)			5	1.916	ns
9	7.6	6.9			
10	32.5	28.9			
11	35.9	35.8			
12	19.8	23.9			
13 and older	4.3	4.4			
Gender			1	.002	ns
Female	51.4	51.6			
Male	48.6	48.4			
Parents Divorced			2	9.580	.008
Yes	46.3	35.0			
No	43.3	58.1			
Don't Know	10.4	6.9			
Race			3	22.791	.001
Hispanic	35.8	21.8			
Black	37.7	58.9			
White	14.5	7.4			
Other	11.9	11.9			
School Grades			4	2.976	ns
Excellent	31.3	25.6			
Very Good	8.2	18.8			
Good	40.7	41.9			
Not Good	8.5	12.5			
Poor	1.3	1.2			

with a mean of 4.41, whereas control participants scored 4.21, $t(485) = 1.94$, $p < .053$ (two-tailed).

Not surprisingly, no differences were found for substance use association or participant alcohol and drug use. At pretest, youths' mean age was 10.83 years; at posttest, approximately 9 months later, their mean age was 11.59 years. Though these young ages are desirable for targeting alcohol and substance use prevention programs, detecting behavior change among early adolescents is difficult. The frequency of substance abuse behavior is low. Behavioral outcomes on the effectiveness of the CD-ROM intervention are not expected until subsequent follow-up measures.

Qualitative. As a result of random assignment, some collaborating sites had higher functioning computers than others. No site was expelled

FIGURE 1. Pretest to Posttest Gain Series: Intervention and Control Arms

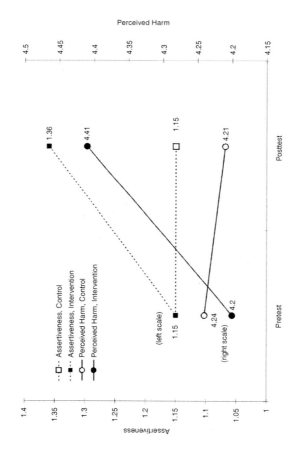

Perceived Harm

Assertiveness

- ☐ - Assertiveness, Control
- ■ - Assertiveness, Intervention
- ○ - Perceived Harm, Control
- ● - Perceived Harm, Intervention

(left scale)

(right scale)

Pretest

Posttest

1.36

4.41

1.15

4.21

1.15

4.24

4.2

from the study based on computer quality. Complications arose at less than one-third of the 26 intervention sites. In these instances, the existing RAM (Random Access Memory) on the computers was insufficient for adequate interaction with the CD-ROM. The necessary upgrades in RAM were arranged, and this gift fostered a positive relationship with agency staff.

Once the appropriate platform was achieved, SODAS City met with enthusiasm from collaborating sites, parents, and youths. Site staff appeared to value the ease with which they could implement the intervention and often asked if they could provide the game to youths who were not in the study (which was possible because of the randomized block design that assigned sites to arms). After the 10 sessions were delivered, several site directors asked to enroll incoming youths into the program (which was not possible because of the absence of consent and baseline data). As a result of their positive experiences with the software, site staff have requested other types of CD-ROM interventions when they become available.

Uniformly positive feedback has come from youth participants in the intervention arm. Of the 329 participants, only three youths attrited. At sites, youths were enthusiastic about interacting with the CD-ROM; often staff had to ensure that no more than one episode was played per session. Over the intervention delivery period, the investigators received a number of telephone calls from youths wondering when they were to receive additional program content. Several requested that SODAS City be sent home to sisters, brothers, and friends.

DISCUSSION AND CONCLUSIONS

Modest findings from this feasibility study suggest that new technologies, specifically CD-ROM technology, hold promise for transmitting alcohol abuse prevention program content to high-risk youths. Through interactive skills-based sessions, participants in the intervention arm showed an increased understanding of assertiveness. Youths practiced being assertive and witnessed the benefits of assertion through simulated real-life scenarios.

The data suggest that youths who interacted with the 10-session CD-ROM were more cognizant of the harmful effects of alcohol. Again, this message was gained through interactive play rather than passive listening. Given multiple opportunities to see the negative consequences of using alcohol, intervention participants moved in the desired outcome direction; control participants' measured perceived harm of alcohol remained unchanged.

The positive trends in intervention participants' assertion skills and perceived harm of alcohol are protective factors to help children and adolescents avoid problems with alcohol and other substance use. Assertion skills help youths to distinguish among assertive, aggressive, and passive behaviors while increasing their social proficiency and resiliency. With respect to decisions regarding alcohol and substance use, youths with an increased perception of the harm of alcohol and increased assertiveness are more likely to make decisions away from alcohol and drug use.

The lack of change in alcohol and substance use between intervention and control arms was somewhat disappointing. But the absence of behavior change is understandable and arguably appropriate, considering the low base rates of drinking and substance use among members of the young sample at pretest and in light of the close proximity of posttesting to intervention. Because study participants were from urban areas, generalization of any findings to all American youths is unwarranted.

Despite these limitations, the study has strengths. During 10 interactive sessions, youths rehearsed real-life situations, experienced the consequences of poor decision making, and compared those results with the outcomes of better decision making. High-quality graphics, attention to cultural nuances and challenging yet age-appropriate objectives ensured successful engagement with the participants. The use of CD-ROM technology was feasible for delivering alcohol abuse prevention material. Study sites implemented the program quickly and easily, without burdensome materials and labor intensive training.

For schools and social service agencies, time and money are precious commodities. Effective prevention programs that can be implemented without depleting resources will likely be preferred to programs that are costly and time-consuming. The portability of our CD-ROM was helpful when participants moved or stopped attending their afterschool program. When these displaced youths gained access to a computer, they could participate fully in the research, receiving intervention identical to other participants. Although initial development and creative costs were high, the final program was duplicated and packaged for less than $1.00 per child.

Additional work with CD-ROM technology in the field of alcohol abuse and other prevention science is warranted. Investigators must and will continue to use the latest tools available to reach target youths with effective programs. Doubtless, we will observe the development of interactive prevention programs online in the future. Until Internet accessibility is pervasive and content is not limited by bandwidth, prevention should continue to explore the exciting and aforementioned advantages of CD-ROM technology. Perhaps the present research will aid in that exploration.

REFERENCES

Botvin, G. J., Baker, E., Dusenbury, L. D., Botvin, E. M., & Diaz, T. (1995). Long-term follow-up results of a randomized drug abuse prevention trial in a White middle-class population. *Journal of the American Medical Association, 273,* 1106-1112.

Botvin, G. J., Baker, E., Dusenbury, L., Tortu, S., & Botvin, E. M. (1990). Preventing adolescent drug abuse through a multimodal cognitive-behavioral approach: Results of a 3-year study. *Journal of Consulting & Clinical Psychology, 58,* 437-446.

Botvin, G. J., Epstein, J. A., Baker, E., Diaz, T., & Ifill-Williams, M. (1997). School-based drug abuse prevention with inner-city minority youths. *Journal of Child & Adolescent Substance Abuse, 6,* 5-19.

Botvin, G. J., & Kantor, L. W. (2000). Preventing alcohol and tobacco use through life skills training. *Alcohol Health & Research World, 24,* 250-257.

Centers for Disease Control and Prevention. (2001). Youth 2001 Online: Alcohol/Other Drug Use. In *Youth Risk Behavior Surveillance System.* Retrieved July 30, 2002, from http://apps.nccd.cdc.gov/YRBSS/GraphV.asp

Centers for Disease Control and Prevention. (2000). Youth Risk Behavior Surveillance–United States, 1999. *Morbidity and Mortality Weekly Report: CDC Surveillance Summaries 49*(No. SS-5) 1-94.

Deluty, R. H. (1984). Behavioral validation of the Children's Action Tendency Scale. *Journal of Behavioral Assessment, 6,* 115-130.

Deluty, R. H. (1979). Children's Action Tendency Scale: A self-reported measure of aggressiveness, assertiveness, and submissiveness in children. *Journal of Consulting and Clinical Psychology, 47,* 1061-1071.

Digital Divide Network. (2002). *Digital Divide Basics.* Retrieved July 31, 2002, from http://www.digitaldividenetwork.org/content/sections/index.cfm?key=2

Grant, B. F., & Dawson, D. A. (1997). Age at onset of alcohol use and association with DSM-IV alcohol abuse and dependence: Results from the National Longitudinal Alcohol Epidemiologic Survey. *Journal of Substance Abuse, 9,* 103-110.

Hawkins, J. D., Catalano, R. F., Kosterman, R., Abbott, R., & Hill, K. G. (1999). Preventing adolescent health-risk behaviors by strengthening protection during childhood. *Archives of Pediatric & Adolescent Medicine, 153,* 226-234.

Johnston, L. D., O'Malley, P. M., & Bachman, J. G. (2002). *Monitoring the Future national results on adolescent drug use: Overview of key findings, 2001.* Rockville, MD: National Institute on Drug Abuse.

National Cancer Institute. (1991). *Cancer among blacks and other minorities: Statistical profiles.* Bethesda, MD: U.S. Department of Health and Human Services.

National Institute on Alcohol Abuse and Alcoholism. (1998). Drinking in the United States: Main Findings from the 1992 National Longitudinal Alcohol Epidemiologic Survey (NLAES). In *US Alcohol Epidemiologic Data Reference Manual* (Vol. 6). Bethesda, MD: Author.

Rotheram-Borus, M. J. (2000). Expanding the range of interventions to reduce HIV among adolescents. *AIDS, 14*(Suppl. 1), S33-S40.

Scheier, L., Botvin, G. J., & Griffin, K. W. (2001). Preventive intervention effects on developmental progression in drug use: Structural equation modeling analyses using longitudinal data. *Prevention Science, 2*(2), 91-112.

Schinke, S. P., Botvin, G. J., & Orlandi, M. A. (1991). *Substance abuse in children and adolescents.* Newbury Park, CA: Sage Publications.

Schinke, S. P., Gordon, A. N., & Weston, R. E. (1990). Self-instruction to prevent HIV infection among African-American and Hispanic-American Adolescents. *Journal of Consulting and Clinical Psychology, 58,* 432-436.

U.S. Department of Commerce, Economics and Statistics Administration National Telecommunications and Information Administration. (2002, February). *A Nation Online: How Americans Are Expanding Their Use of the Internet.* Retrieved July 27, 2002, from http://www.ntia.doc.gov/ntiahome/dn/

U.S. Department of Health and Human Services. (2000). *The 2000HHS Poverty Guidelines.* Retrieved July 28, 2002, from http://aspe.hhs.gov/poverty/00poverty.htm

Constructing Better Futures via Video

Peter W. Dowrick

Center on Disability Studies
University of Hawaii at Manoa

Beverly I. Tallman
Marilyn E. Connor

Center for Human Development
University of Alaska Anchorage

SUMMARY. Some individuals can rise above disadvantaged environments by cognitively constructing better ones. One way to go beyond limited environments is by creating *video futures*. This article describes applications of video-based futures planning, in which teenagers find meaning in their current educational setting to prepare them for adulthood. We also describe the systematic training of school-based personnel to support the skills and positive attitudes of their students with carefully planned and edited videos that show *future* capability of the in-

Address correspondence to: Prof. Peter W. Dowrick, Center on Disability Studies, 1776 University Avenue UA4-6, Manoa, HI 96822, USA.

The authors would like to thank the many colleagues, school-based personnel, students, and parents who contributed to the progress of Video Futures.

The program development referred to herein was supported in part by U.S. Dept. of Education, Office of Special Education Programs (awds H158K30024, H158V6005). The article was written without financial support by Peter W. Dowrick, based on previous reports and other information.

[Haworth co-indexing entry note]: "Constructing Better Futures via Video." Dowrick, Peter W., Beverly I. Tallman, and Marilyn E. Connor. Co-published simultaneously in *Journal of Prevention & Intervention in the Community* (The Haworth Press, Inc.) Vol. 29, No. 1/2, 2005, pp. 131-144; and: *Technology Applications in Prevention* (ed: Steven Godin) The Haworth Press, Inc., 2005, pp. 131-144. Single or multiple copies of this article are available for a fee from The Haworth Document Delivery Service [1-800-HAWORTH, 9:00 a.m. - 5:00 p.m. (EST). E-mail address: docdelivery@haworthpress.com].

dividual (self modeling and feedforward). We report diverse case studies to illustrate the methodologies, the range of applications, and typical outcomes. Follow-up of dissemination (especially the Video Futures Start-Up Kit) indicates successful replications, particularly in Kentucky and Aotearoa New Zealand. *[Article copies available for a fee from The Haworth Document Delivery Service: 1-800-HAWORTH. E-mail address: <docdelivery@haworthpress. com> Website: <http://www.HaworthPress.com> © 2005 by The Haworth Press, Inc. All rights reserved.]*

KEYWORDS. Video futures, feedforward, disabilities, education, community, transitions

An interesting proposition by Bandura is that there are three types of environments: those that severely delimit people's operating options, those that offer choices, and "created" environments that allow people to become self-determined beyond the apparent limitations of their circumstances (Bandura, 1997, p. 163). For example, Ernie may have one school and one shop to go to, transport choices of Shank's pony (walking) or bus, and one affordable place to live, the current housing complex. At the next, less restrictive level up, Maysie may have multiple educational choices including private piano lessons, the flexibility to shop anywhere in a 30 km radius, getting there by foot, bus, taxi or private car, while living in a private house with options to renovate or move. Joachim, however, lives nowhere defined; nevertheless he sees himself graduating from college, owning a successful business, and beating Tiger Woods at golf, maybe arm wrestling as well. Constructed environments do not give empowerment, but give people such as Joachim life enriching ways to use the power/skills/education/capital they have. And it gives them the belief in using that capital (i.e., self-efficacy; Bandura, 1997).

Considerable applied research has indicated the promise of video self modeling to help the acquisition of skills and attitudes for success (Dowrick, 1999). In this strategy, a provider creates a short (2 min.) video of a person successfully dealing with a normally challenging, even "impossible," situation–for example, a selectively mute child talking to his teacher (Pigott & Gonzales, 1986), a librarian winning the state championship in power lifting (Franks & Maile, 1991). Video self modeling has successfully addressed a range of skills, from communication (e.g., in children with autism; Buggey, Toombs, Gardener, &

Cervetti, 1999) to physical performance (Dowrick & Raeburn, 1995), to mathematics (Schunk & Hanson, 1986), in a range of abilities (e.g., would-be swimmers; Starek & McCullagh, 1999), and ages (e.g., elderly; Neef, Bill-Harvey, Shade, Iezzi, & DeLorenzo, 1995).

Self modeling often provides a collection of best recent efforts, inconsistent exemplars that an individual wishes to achieve more regularly. But many such videos also provide credible illustrations of *successes not yet achieved*–an effect known as *feedforward* (in contrast to feedback; Dowrick, 1983, 1997). Feedforward, creating images of successes yet to be achieved, provides not only a teaching methodology, but a philosophy. It is a philosophy useful in community-responsiveness (Dowrick, Power et al., 2001), especially where the futures are bleak or void in the minds of constituents. Whereas feedforward can be in any medium (audiotape, drawings, role play, imagination), it seems singularly powerful in *video*, which provides compelling, moving images that can be reviewed repeatedly and exactly, as often as required or desired. Because the videos are of oneself, they empower or advance competencies in the culture of the participants.

About 10 years ago we became interested in ways to extend video feedforward to the more distant future and to the issues of training community-based professionals in the practicalities of using these techniques. This article provides highlights of these efforts, which were partially funded for 6 years by the U.S. Office of Special Education Programs.

VIDEO-BASED FUTURES PLANNING

A common approach to helping youth (with disabilities) in high school plan for their transition to adulthood is called *futures planning* (Holburn & Vietze, 2002). It usually involves many discussions with the youth, family, educators, etc., to produce a list of scenarios or objectives around potential jobs or education, living arrangements, and social life. We thought it may be productive to put these scenarios on videotape, with the youth depicting themselves, say 5 years into the future (Dowrick, Tallman, Mercer, & Donnelly, 1993). Principles from video self modeling practice, typically used to teach specific skills for the immediate future, would be incorporated as applicable.

We define *exploration videos* as those that depict a relatively remote potential future (say 6 months to 5 years hence), for an identified individual, group, or community. The videos may be based on a personal futures plan with multiple considerations of someone's life, or on a specific challenging change of environment, such as a new or very different job. The futures plan or desired way to face a challenge may emphasize hopes and dreams as much as reality. Such a video can make a plan extremely tangible–in which the projected future is enacted by the individuals affected, recorded and edited onto videotape. An exploration video may show any alternative vision of the individual's world–perhaps recorded by the person themselves (Ben, Wiedle, Tallman, & Dowrick, 1996).

METHOD

The overall strategy that evolved for video-based futures planning is as follows. It is designed around teenagers with disabilities, but could easily be generalized to other situations.
Main Objective: Develop Lifestyle Images in Key Domains:

- Living arrangements
- Relationship to family
- Social life
- Other recreation
- Employment
- Primary means of transport

Planning Process

For a high school student in special education, a picture is built of what his or her life could look like soon after age 21 or 22. Not only is the beginning of adult life challenging, as it is for most youth, but the mandated systems of support change in ways that seldom provide adequate continuity (Dowrick, 2003). The process includes a series of meetings and activities involving the teenager, parents, teacher, and special educator. Other family members, social worker, counselor, vocational agency personnel, and so on, may be included to the extent they figure significantly in the teen's life.

Video of the Future

The teen has the last say if the contents of future scenarios are disputed (which they usually are). Loose scripts are developed around each target domain. For example, what started originally as "be independent" becomes the identification, say, of wanting to own a car and a drivers license—with the associated costs and lifestyle—and implications for income, job, social life, recreation, and so on. So a scene is planned with Ms. or Mr. T. (the teen) in a parking lot, discussing the price of a motor vehicle, reaching an agreement, receiving the keys, and apparently driving away. The finished video, covering important elements of all six domains, is about 5 minutes long. The videos may promote intermediate objectives. They usually motivate engagement in the educational activities and skills training necessary to meet these objectives. They can be reviewed, referenced, and revised as progress is (or is not) made toward the long-term goals of the transition.

The general steps developing a personal or community responsive video are set out in Table 1. Specific steps for a video with community integration goals are illustrated in the example below.

Case Example

Several Self-Determination classes were held for at-risk youth, with discussions on goal setting, self-efficacy, etc. (Ben, Wiedle, Andersen, & Dowrick, 1995). These youth were offered the opportunity to participate in Video Futures. One of them we will call "Carl." One of our staff helped him to develop a list of hopes and dreams for the future. In discussions with Carl, his family, and others, the list grew to 21 items that could be part of his adulthood. They encompassed the six "key" domains of life, listed with bullets above, for which we considered transition planning to be most important (Dowrick & Wiedle, 1996).

Carl then met with another of our staff, "Cathie," to identify his six to ten most important aspirations. Cathie explained that we would like to make a movie of his future, like science fiction, with him in the starring role. He could also help plan and edit the video. Carl thought it was a cool (if a bit puzzling) idea. To put the items on video, they had to become much more specific and tangible than they were. "Live independently" became "have my own apartment with friends visiting but not living there." That had implications for what type of apartment, to be affordable with the type of job he had identified, and what would you do with friends who came over? If you're going to be "working with cars," will you be fixing them, will you need some classes at college?

Carl and Cathie readily agreed on seven situations (scenarios), with enough specificity for rough scripts or storyboards. Cathie made location arrangements, using her house and car, the mechanics shop at the community college, and permission from the amusement park to film at

TABLE 1. A Six-Step Process for Constructing Better Futures on Video

---

DEVELOPMENT OF "FUTURES" ON VIDEO

1. Conceptualization of the video
    identify the consumers–who needs to be included?
    what challenges will they face, what skills will they need (include expert knowledge)?
    gain collaboration and participation, to set good goals
    assess what's happening now, in behaviorally observable terms
    identify what should be happening, or what the consumers want to happen, likewise

2. Pre-production: script or storyboard
    select the target skills or desired goals
    establish components of what the consumer can already do
    establish resources for film events and locations
    what is desired outcome (think like a human/community services professional)?
    how could that be shown (think like a movie director)?
    write a script (shot list) or draw a storyboard, scene by scene

3. Production: filming the "capture" footage
    talk over each scene, on location; suggest and demonstrate what to do
    rehearse once, then film with cues and prompts, external support if necessary
    check the footage and the sound; film again if necessary
    select camera angles, backgrounds, and do the next scene, until finished the scenario

4. Post-production: editing the video
    review the capture tape; copy all that's needed to the hard drive (if computer editing available)
    identify and document desired footage (trim each scene, if on computer)
    edit by copying, resequencing, repeating selected segments from one VCR to another (or with suitable software, such as iMovie2)
    check the edited version against the plan (storyboard), and copy for the consumer (usually VHS or CD-ROM)

5. Viewing, following a schedule
    for skills training, arrange three or more times a week for 2 weeks
    for video explorations, plan for once per week/month, take to planning meetings, etc.
    write a schedule of planned dates for viewing
    assign responsible person to record actual dates and reactions to viewing

6. Evaluation: based on progress data, reassing the goals
    monitor behaviors, attitudes, and related events
    follow up, and determine a plan for the future

the go-kart circuit. With other students we frequently used the local supermarkets, travel agents, university facilities (restaurant, vacant student housing, etc.) and the fronts of buildings: banks, churches, Division of Motor Vehicles, and so on. Each filming session was individually planned for no more than five short shots, to be edited into 30-40 seconds of tape, per scenario. Sometimes they took a videographer with them, otherwise James did the camera and directed the action.

It took 2 weeks to arrange locations and collect the footage necessary for editing. Carl watched Cathie's first cut with him, to approve or make any suggestions for changes, and he helped to choose a little background music. The final edit of seven situations was 6 minutes long, including titles with Alaskan scenery and credits at the end showing Carl as the producer and owner of the tape.

Creating Futures in Early Adulthood

Twenty teenagers in a special high school program for students at risk took part in this program referred to as Video Futures (Dowrick & Skouge, 2001). All these students had disabilities with special education classifications of some type. Many of the students had medical conditions or judicial records considered to put them at additional risk.

About 40 students in the program were introduced to self-determination in the classroom, and they undertook personal futures planning with their families. Along lines similar to those illustrated by Carl above, 20 youth, ages 16-19 years, accepted an option to make a video (Ben, Wiedle, Tallman, & Dowrick, 1996). All these videos included topics to represent most or all of the six specific domains as listed above, depending on individual student preferences. All goals were chosen within the six domains, but some students chose two of one and none of another.

Thirteen students listed some type of course or class among their goals, and virtually half of them chose a second learning goal. Most popular among all students was culinary arts, often including interest to work as a chef; second for girls was early childhood development. Thirteen youth also identified living in a house or apartment independently of their parents as a goal for their video. Other popular choices were getting a driver's license and/or buying a car–no other modes of transport were chosen.

Of these 20 students, 5 transferred to other places before the end of high school. Five years later, the other 15 are considered by their previous school administrator to have made successful transitions to adult life–more successful than comparable cohorts who did not participate in video futures (G. Donnelly, personal communication, 27 Nov. 2002). Many have fulfilled some of their video goals/dreams: getting jobs, taking college classes, getting driving licenses, living in apartments. One young woman lived for 2 years in an apartment then bought her own home under a special program from Housing and Urban Development. She was also featured at a vocational conference for her work reliability and initiative; prior to her video, her parents had expressed their expectation that she would never leave home or work full time. Ten individuals participated in the 1999 International People First Conference, where they presented on their experiences in transition and self-determination. They were interviewed (on camera; Ben, Caires, Connor, & Dowrick, 1999), and all spoke enthusiastically about their new hopes and dreams, emphasizing travel, better employment, and families.

The overall outcomes for the students in the video-based futures program were above the expectation for students of their classification in the school system. It is not an objective, let alone an expectation, that the goals/dreams expressed in videos would necessarily be achieved as depicted. It is the belief in the possibility not the inevitability that allows the creation of positive futures, or constructed environments. Individuals may never own that business or travel the world, but as with other aspirational goal setting (Bandura, 1997), the realistic pursuit of those images can lead to a greater engagement with life.

TRAINING EDUCATORS AND OTHER COMMUNITY PERSONNEL

The video-based futures planning and other exploration videos have significant community impact in that they promote a higher level of community participation than might otherwise be expected. We sought to take these possibilities to a higher level by developing a system of training community-based personnel to apply a wide range of video futures techniques in their locations. Aside from key individuals who were trained, the most important outcome was the development of a *Video Futures Start-Up Kit* (Dowrick, Connor, and associates, 1999), essentially a self-teaching package for aspiring providers.

Establishing the Training Needs, Working with Educators

We spent a year working in collaboration with seven school-based personnel in two districts. They included teachers, special educators, speech therapists, and vocational educators. Our university-based (grant-funded) staff provided video self modeling or other "positive video" type implementations, with the school staff in apprenticeship roles. Some were very successful. For example, one vocational teacher decided to make a class project of making self model videos of mock job interview situations. He claimed later that the year's exit interviews and actual job applications and placements were the best ever for his class.

In the meantime, we took very careful notes about the knowledge/skills strengths/barriers for the school personnel to become independent providers of video futures.

Direct Training, Development of More Materials

The next year, we trained 14 personnel, including some non-profit agency staff. This time our staff directly supervised the "apprentices," giving them responsibility for storyboards, videotaping, and editing under our guidance. We developed a curriculum (Connor, 1999), obtained approval for one credit of continuing education, and offered it again the next year to another 14 individuals. That, of course, stimulated the gathering of print and video teaching materials.

Evaluation of the Training System, Evolution of the Video Futures Start-Up Kit

The 1-credit course was evaluated positively by participants (av. 4.6 on 5-pt. scale). All individuals produced videos in the course, and about half subsequently made videos for their students/consumers. We now offer half-day, full-day, or 2-day workshops to achieve similar outcomes.

Of enduring interest is the emerging training package. The production of someone's future on video can be identified in six steps:

1. Conceptualization of the video, based on knowledge of the methodology and working with the consumer to set goals.
2. Pre-production: script or storyboard.
3. Production: videotaping the "capture" footage.
4. Post-production: editing the video.

5. Viewing, following a schedule.
6. Evaluation: based on progress data, reassessing the goals.

These steps can be discretely taught, and thus provide the elements of the training system. The User's Guide (75-pg. manual) lays out these elements, plus examples and technical tips for videography (Dowrick & Meunier, 1999). A graduate student employed in the grant improved and evaluated the guide for his thesis. Four videotapes were produced: (1) an introduction, including faces and voices of participants; (2) a six-step (how-to) illustration of the procedure; (3) vignettes from applications produced by trainees of the system; and (4) examples of video-based futures planning.

Speech and Language Example

One of the star trainees was "Ms. Jenn." She created five videos in quick succession, and became a mentor for other speech therapists. Here is one example from her casebook.

Concept. "Deb" was an 18-year-old whose rapid and slurred speech was hard to understand. Most people could understand only 50% of what she said, so her goal was to raise that to 90%. Despite clinic-based therapy, her community-based speech had not improved in some months. She was positive about the prospects of video self modeling.

Pre-Production. Ms. Jenn could improve Deb's speech intelligibility to 95% but only in the clinic and for short periods. Together they planned an opening for the video, some phrases to illustrate various words and vowels for improved intelligibility (which they rehearsed), and a positive ending.

Production. Ms. Jenn recorded the opening and the ending. When Deb rehearsed a phrase to criterion, Ms. Jenn recorded two or three examples, until all phrases were captured.

Post-Production. Ms. Jenn copied the segments of video she wanted onto another tape, laying down the opening, followed by the best example of the first phrase, and so on. She also dubbed some applause onto the sound track at the end of each phrase.

Viewing. Deb viewed her self modeling video at the clinic three times a week for 2 weeks, during which she reported enjoying seeing herself being successful on video. She took the video home and watched it occasionally to prevent lapses in her intelligibility.

Evaluation. After 2 weeks, her intelligibility improved to 90% in the community, according to observations by the therapist. A week later it reached 95% and was maintained throughout the school year. No other teenage students receiving services for intelligibility without self modeling in the clinic achieved comparable results.

This type of feedforward intervention fits the category of *transferring behaviors across settings* (one of seven categories, identified by Dowrick, 1999). That is, a skill or behavior readily achieved in one setting (exclusively) can be achieved in other situations, simply by viewing a video that shows the behavior, probably not necessarily showing the other setting. Ms. Jenn, normally shy in public settings herself, presented this case at a school district meeting of speech and language pathologists. Two more of her examples appear in the Vignettes video of the Start-Up Kit: a boy improving articulation of a specific consonant, and a youth asking for directions.

Vocational Education Examples

Other stars of the program were "Mr. George" and "Ms. Gay Lee." Their interventions helped improve quality of life in the community and the workplace for several individuals. Here is an example of *personal safety*—staying safe in public places.

Concepts. "Carrie" was a 17-year-old with Asperger's syndrome. She felt susceptible to harassment, especially by the sexual comments of one male high school student. She asked Mr. George for help. Together they decided to make a feedforward video of appropriate assertiveness skills.

Pre-Production. Carrie and Mr. George brainstormed some assertive phrases and wrote them down. They decided on five scenarios and the sequence of them.

Production. One of Carrie's male friends agreed to role play the offender. They rehearsed the scenes and Carrie became very enthusiastic. Mr. George videotaped each scene after it had been practiced, placing the camera behind Carrie's friend so she could be seen clearly while he was obscured and unidentifiable.

Post-Production. A week later, Mr. George copied the most effectively assertive scenes onto another tape, adding an opening title and end credits.

Viewing. After editing was complete, Carrie watched the video twice. She arranged a schedule to return and view the tape eight times over the next 2 weeks.

Evaluation. Mr. George had arranged self-reporting by Carrie before, during, and after videotaping. The first day after editing and viewing the tape, Carrie reported she did not expect to need it any more. She had, without difficulty, told the offending student to leave her alone. He had apologized–and asked to be her friend. Given that Mr. George had delayed a week before editing, it appears that viewing the tape, not just role playing, had been effective in her case.

This example fits the self modeling category of *transferring role play to the real world* (Dowrick, 1999), for which video (and possibly audio recording) seems uniquely advantageous.

Other Examples. "Edward" was a 19-year-old with a cognitive disability. On his job training site, he would avoid (escape) supervisor requests by saying "but I'm doing such-and-such right now." Ms. Gay Lee helped him by creating a self modeling video, including four different responses, ranging from "sure, I'll do it right now," to "let me just finish packing these shelves, it'll only take 10 minutes." Edward's supervisor helped with the script and role plays for the video. After watching the video every day for 2 weeks, Edward completely stopped saying "but I'm doing such-and-such right now," substituting more appropriate responses, without losing his (desirable) assertiveness.

"Dorothy" was a 13-year-old who used a wheelchair, and had begun work experience in the community. Her parents were concerned about her safety in catching the bus. Dorothy and Mr. George scripted and filmed a video of her catching the bus, having enjoyable but not risky conversations with passengers, nor accepting rides from strangers while waiting for the bus. Getting on and off the bus was recorded on location, and the strangers were role played in a school room by classmates.

Dorothy viewed the tape at least once a day for two weeks. Before, during, and after the self modeling, Mr. George followed the bus in his car every day to provide help if necessary. Within the two-week viewing period, Dorothy was able to use the bus without assistance. Four months later, she and her parents reported that she frequently used public transportation and they all felt comfortable about it.

FUTURE DIRECTIONS

About 50 sites have adopted Video Futures nationally and internationally (England, Canada, New Zealand, Australia, with expressions of interest in Korea, Germany, and other countries). Many agencies made agreements to provide anecdotes and data. So far, the most reliable reports have come from Kentucky, New Zealand, and Australia, in addition to Alaska where the Start-Up Kit was developed. Although some sites report difficulty related to equipment and cooperation, the outcomes have been in line with the cases described above: widely successful and sometimes extremely rapid with unexpected generalization and maintenance. Users find the system challenging because they have to think like movie directors, a new skill for most. They also find it rewarding and enjoyable. Feedforward is arguably the least restrictive intervention in that it is forward-looking and focuses entirely on positive outcomes, rather than backward-looking attempting to correct errors.

These examples emphasize community applications. They involve individuals, families, or small groups, and facilitate more meaningful engagement in the world. There are obvious extensions to this approach. For example, an entire community could be involved in the production of a video of their future. It could be a neighborhood or town. Or it could be a sub-community, such a gang or an association of professors. They could collaborate to plan, film, and edit a video of their community 5 to 10 years into the future–balancing, as did the youth with disabilities, their hopes and dreams with reality. Then they could show it for public discussion or to legislators (like at an IEP meeting). It would provide an interesting contrast to other community-change videos, which have also proved effective (Henny, 1983) but tend to highlight the community's woes as much as their solutions. It is certainly an interesting prospect that we look forward to addressing, or hearing about from others who may take up this prospect.

REFERENCES

Bandura, A. (1997). *Self-efficacy: The exercise of control.* New York: Freeman.

Ben, K., Caires, J., Connor, M.E., & Dowrick, P.W. (1999). *Video futures: A new frontier.* Anchorage, AK: Center for Human Development, University of Alaska Anchorage [video].

Ben, K., Wiedle, J., Andersen, C., & Dowrick, P.W. (1995). *Fostering self-determination: Activities, lessons, resources.* Anchorage, AK: Center for Human Development, University of Alaska Anchorage.

Ben, K., Wiedle, J., Tallman, B.I., & Dowrick, P.W. (1996). *Increasing skills necessary for self-determination through video based personal futures planning: Final report.* Washington, DC: U.S. Office of Special Education Programs.

Buggey, T., Toombs, K., Gardener, P., & Cervetti, M. (1999). Training responding behaviors in students with autism: Using videotaped self modeling. *Journal of Positive Behavior Interventions, 1,* 205-214.

Connor, M.E. (1999). *Video futures: Interventions for school and community.* Curriculum approved by Anchorage School District, Alaska.

Dowrick, P.W. (1983). Self modelling. In P.W. Dowrick & S.J. Biggs (Eds.), *Using video: Psychological and social applications* (pp. 105-124). Chichester, UK: Wiley.

Dowrick, P.W. (1997). Video feedforward. *Northeast Healthcare Management* (June), pp. 6-9.

Dowrick, P.W. (1999). A review of self modeling and related interventions. *Applied and Preventive Psychology, 8,* 23-39.

Dowrick, P.W. (2003). Preventing school drop out. In T. Gullotta & M. Bloom (Eds.), *Encyclopedia of Primary Prevention. Section III: Adolescence.*

Dowrick, P.W., Connor, M.E., and associates. (1999). *The Video Futures Start-Up Kit.* Anchorage: Center for Human Development: UCE.

Dowrick, P.W., & Meunier, R. (1999). *Video futures: A guide to self modeling and related procedures* (2nd ed.). Honolulu: Center on Disability Studies, University of Hawaii.

Dowrick, P.W., Power, T.J., Manz, P.H., Ginsburg-Block, M., Leff, S.S., & Kim-Rupnow, W.S. (2001). Community responsiveness: Examples from under-resourced urban schools. *Journal of Prevention & Intervention in the Community, 21,* 71-90.

Dowrick, P.W., & Raeburn, J.M. (1995). Self-modeling: Rapid skill training for children with physical disabilities. *Journal of Developmental and Physical Disabilities, 7,* 25-37.

Dowrick, P.W., & Skouge, J. (2001). Creating video futures: Potential of video empowerment in postsecondary education. *Disability Studies Quarterly, 21,* 59-76.

Dowrick, P.W., Tallman, B.I., Mercer, M., & Donnelly, G. (1993). *Increasing skills necessary for self-determination through video based personal futures planning.* Grant funded by U.S. Department of Education, Office of Special Education Programs, 1993-96.

Franks, I.M., & Maile, L.J. (1991). The use of video in sport skill acquisition. In P.W. Dowrick & associates, *Practical guide to using video in the behavioral sciences.* New York: Wiley Interscience.

Henny, L. (1983). Video in the community. In P.W. Dowrick & S.J. Biggs (Eds.), *Using video: Psychological and social applications* (pp. 167-177). Chichester, UK: Wiley.

Holburn, S., & Vietze, P.M. (Eds.). (2002). *Person-centered planning: Research, practice, and future directions.* Baltimore: Brookes.

Neef, N.A., Bill-Harvey, D., Shade, D., Iezzi, M., & DeLorenzo, T. (1995). Exercise participation with videotaped modeling effects on balance and gait in elderly residents of care facilities. *Behavior Therapy, 26,* 135-151.

Pigott, H.E., & Gonzales, F.P. (1987). The efficacy of videotape self-modeling to treat an electively mute child. *Journal of Clinical Child Psychology, 16,* 106-110.

Schunk, D.H., & Hanson, A.R. (1989). Self-modeling and children's cognitive skill learning. *Journal of Educational Psychology, 81,* 155-163.

Starek, J., & McCullagh, P. (1999). The effect of self modeling on the performance of beginning swimmers. *The Sport Psychologist, 13,* 269-287.

General Characteristics
of Internet Use Among Health Educators:
Implications for the Profession

Kelli McCormack Brown
Jane Ellery

University of South Florida
College of Public Health

Paula Perlmutter

Hunter College Center on AIDS,
Drugs and Community Health

SUMMARY. The Internet plays an important role in health education today. This study attempts to fill a void in the literature regarding Internet use, including motivators and barriers for health educators. Using a modified version of the Total Design Method, a survey concerning Internet use was mailed to a stratified random sample of 1559 health educators in the United States. Seven-hundred thirty-eight surveys were usable for a 55% response rate. Descriptive statistics were calculated for all variables, and

---

Address correspondence to: Kelli McCormack Brown, Associate Professor, University of South Florida, College of Public Health, 13201 Bruce B. Downs Boulevard, Tampa, FL 33612-3805 (E-mail: kmbrown@hsc.usf.edu).

This study was partially funded by the University of South Florida Research Council.

[Haworth co-indexing entry note]: "General Characteristics of Internet Use Among Health Educators: Implications for the Profession." Brown, Kelli McCormack, Jane Ellery, and Paula Perlmutter. Co-published simultaneously in *Journal of Prevention & Intervention in the Community* (The Haworth Press, Inc.) Vol. 29, No. 1/2, 2005, pp. 145-159; and: *Technology Applications in Prevention* (ed: Steven Godin) The Haworth Press, Inc., 2005, pp. 145-159. Single or multiple copies of this article are available for a fee from The Haworth Document Delivery Service [1-800-HAWORTH, 9:00 a.m. - 5:00 p.m. (EST). E-mail address: docdelivery@haworthpress.com].

145

exploratory factor analyses were performed on three domains of questions from the survey. Adequate access, relative advantage and problems with Web sites are factors that influence Internet use among health educators. The majority of respondents had access to the Internet at home and work, and over two-thirds used e-mail daily. Implications for the health education profession are provided. *[Article copies available for a fee from The Haworth Document Delivery Service: 1-800-HAWORTH. E-mail address: <docdelivery@haworthpress.com> Website: <http://www.HaworthPress.com> © 2005 by The Haworth Press, Inc. All rights reserved.]*

KEYWORDS. Internet, health education, barriers, access, training

INTRODUCTION

The Internet is the most popular computer network in the world. It has approximately 250 million users worldwide, a number estimated to increase to more than 765 million by year-end 2005 (Computer Industry Almanac, 1999). Powell and Clarke (2002) report over 3 billion Web documents available, with at least 2% of these sites health related. Not only has this technology penetrated both home and work environments, it has now become essential for educators (Jackson & Chun-Ju Chang, 2001). The Internet now plays an important role in health education, too, not only as a valuable information resource, but also a vehicle for enhanced health education programs in schools, hospitals, community health centers, and worksites, in addition to continuing their professional training. The Internet has allowed health professionals and consumers access to information they never dreamed imaginable, information that formerly was prohibitively difficult to retrieve.

The Internet is always open and online information is readily available. Although the Internet appears to be gaining popularity on a wide scale, a lack of information still exists regarding its use among health educators. How can health educators effectively use the Internet for prevention of STDs, cancer, and other diseases, and for promotion of healthful eating, physical activity and other desired health practices? How will online continuing education offerings benefit health educators? Moreover, if health educators are not currently using the Internet, what are the barriers standing in their way, and what can be done to help motivate them to adopt its use? Despite the fact that articles have been written for health educators describing how to use the Internet to obtain reliable information (McCormack Brown, 2001; McCormack Brown, 1998; Kotecki & Siegel, 1997), enhance teaching in the classroom (Perrin & Mayhew, 2000; Randolfi, 1998), to support and improve research (Pealer & Weiler, 2000; Kittleson, 1999; Turner & Turner, 1998), conduct needs assessments (Fulop, Loop-Bartick, & Rossett, 1997), and collect data (Reneau et al., 2000; Nicholson et al., 1999; Nicholson et al., 1998), little has been published on assessing the Internet needs of those working in health education settings or approaches to meet those needs (Hollander & Martin, 1999). The purpose of this study was to identify current practices, beliefs, and perceived barriers and motivators with respect to Internet use, and to identify possible strategies for promoting the use of the Internet among health educators.

METHODS

Methods included the development and pilot testing of the *Internet Use: Attitudes and Behaviors Among Health Educators* survey, a stratified random sampling of health educators, and multiple structured mailings of the survey to increase response rate. The Institutional Review Board (IRB) for the University of South Florida approved the study prior to survey implementation.

Survey Development

A draft survey was developed from reviewing the literature of similar surveys concerned with Internet use, beliefs, and behaviors. Survey content addressed use of the Internet among health educators, including motivators and deterrents. The first iteration of the survey consisted of 25 questions. An expert panel, comprised of six individuals involved in Internet technology, health education, academia, and/or survey development, reviewed the survey for content validity (McKenzie, Wood, Kotecki, Clark, & Brey, 1999). For each question, the expert panel was asked to indicate: (1) if the question was appropriate or inappropriate as stated, (2) if the question was clearly stated, and (3) if the response options were adequate or inadequate. The survey was revised according to remarks made by the panel. Whereas some questions were discarded, others were added to achieve the objectives of this study. The final survey consisted of eight sections: (1) Use and Access; (2) Training; (3) Organizational Support and Barriers; (4) Barriers to Internet

Use; (5) Technology Use Behavior; (6) Confidence in Using the Internet; (7) Beliefs About Internet Use; and (8) Demographics.

The format of the questions varied according to subject matter. Some domains employed Likert-type items, whereas others used a close-ended response option. When content decisions were concluded, the survey was re-formatted into a booklet-style survey and coded to be delivered using the Internet. At the suggestion of the expert reviewers, one page of the survey included definitions to assist respondents with difficult or unknown terminology used in the survey (e.g., Internet, Web-based, web-enhanced).

Pilot Testing

The pilot test refers to a set of procedures used by researchers with a small group of subjects to simulate the study that is to be implemented in the future (McDermott & Sarvela, 1999). The purpose of this pilot test was to detect any problems in the data collection instrument, data collection procedures, and data analysis procedures. This step enabled the researchers to correct any problems before the project was implemented on a large scale.

Pre-pilot testing entailed conducting a test-retest in two classes of health education graduate students. Pre-pilot test participants (N = 35) were given the survey at two different times one week apart to determine test-retest reliability. A paired-samples t-test (p < .05) was conducted on the results of each question. Only two questions were found to be statistically significantly different (p = .011 and p = .000). These two questions were revised on the final survey, which consisted of 32 questions.

The second round of pilot testing, conducted with both electronic mail and U.S. mail recipients, took place to determine the effectiveness of the three delivery methods (see Data Collection section). A random sample (n = 60) was generated from the Society for Public Health Education (SOPHE) directory, and placed into one of the three methods of delivery. The overall response rate for all three groups was 28.3% with only one mailing.

Sampling Description

By combining the lists of Certified Health Education Specialists and the Health Education Directory (HEDIR) in October 1999, there were a total of 6499 health educators in all 50 states and the District of Columbia. Five regions were identified (Table 1).

TABLE 1. Stratified Random Sampling

	Region 1	Region 2	Region 3	Region 4	Region 5	Total
Total in Region	1881	1362	1452	473	1331	6499
% of Total	29%	21%	22%	8%	20%	100%
# Surveyed	432	348	369	126	285	1560

Based on an effect size of .20, a confidence interval of 95%, and a power of 90% the total needed per cell is 130 (Kraemer & Thiemann, 1987). Oversampling by a factor of four brought the final total to 520 per cell, and a total of 1559 eligible individuals were surveyed (due to a postal error one survey did not get mailed). The potential participants were stratified by planned method of delivery and by region. Once stratified, the sample from each group was randomly generated using a computer-generated random table of numbers following a simple random sample method without replacement (McDermott & Sarvela, 1999).

Data Collection

The questionnaire was administered using a modified version of the Tailored Design Method (Dillman, 2000). The Tailored Design Method is based on a series of contacts with potential respondents strategically designed to maximize the quality and quantity of responses.

Three methods of survey delivery were utilized for this study. One-third of the potential participants in the sample were invited to participate using a traditional paper and pencil survey format delivered by the postal service, and one-third were invited to participate using electronic mail (e-mail) notification. Both of these groups received a letter from the principal investigator that included the purpose of the survey, a statement that the survey was both confidential and voluntary, the approval number from the IRB, a statement that participants did not need to answer questions that they were uncomfortable with, an approximation of the length of time required to complete the survey, and information on how to receive a copy of the survey results. Additionally, the paper survey group received a survey booklet and a self-addressed stamped (SASE) to return the survey booklet, whereas the e-mail notification group received a link to the Website where the survey was available for them to complete electronically. The final one-third of potential participants received a postcard notifying them of the Website where they could access a copy of the letter from the principal investigator.

This site also linked them to the electronic survey. As with the paper survey group, this postcard was delivered by the postal service.

The two groups that received their original notification through the postal service (the paper and the postcard groups) also received follow-up notifications through the postal service. The remaining group received all communication electronically. Ten days after the initial mailing, all persons who had not responded received a reminder postcard, either electronically or through the postal service, requesting that they complete and return their surveys. Four weeks after the initial notification, all subjects who had not responded received a follow-up mailing that was similar to the initial mailing, including letters and surveys as outlined for the initial mailing. These procedures were used to help ensure the highest rate of response within the time and financial constraints of the study.

Data Analysis

The final survey was administered using a cross-sectional study design. Data coding and entry were facilitated by SPSS 8.0. Descriptive statistics were calculated for all variables, and exploratory factor analyses were performed on three item domains. In each of the factor analysis groups, principal axis factoring was used to extract factors followed by a promax (oblique) rotation to determine a final solution. Four criteria were considered in the determination of the number of meaningful factors to retain for rotation interpretation. These included: eigen values of 1.0, a scree plot, the proportion of variance accounted for, and interpretability (Hatcher, 1994). In the interpretation of the rotated solution, an item was considered to have loaded on the factor if the pattern loading (rotated factor pattern) was 0.4 or greater for the factor and less than 0.4 for all remaining factors (Hatcher, 1994).

RESULTS

Of the 1559 surveys, 212 were returned undeliverable (14%) and 11 were returned without data, resulting in a usable sample of 1336. Among deliverable surveys, 738 surveys were returned for a 55% response rate. The majority of respondents were female (82%), and had at least a master's degree (79%). Many worked in a college/university academic department (23%) or federal/state agency (14%). More than 8 of 10 (84%) had access to the Internet at home or work, 86% used e-mail on 5 or more days each week, and nearly two-thirds (64%) used the Internet on 5 or more days each week (Table 2).

TABLE 2. Demographics of Health Educators and Internet Use* (n = 738)

Gender (n = 719)	Female	82% (590)
	Male	18% (129)
Age (n = 693)	Age Range	22-77 years of age
	Mean Age	41 years of age
Work Setting (n = 707)	College/UniversityAcademic Dept.	23% (160)
	Federal/State Agency	14% (96)
	Hospital	12% (81)
	Nonprofit Agency	10% (75)
	Local Government	8% (59)
	College/University Health Center	7% (51)
	Consultant	6% (43)
	School (K-12)	3% (24)
Highest Degree (n = 717)	Doctorate	22% (159)
	Master's	57% (409)
	Baccalaureate	19% (137)
Internet Access (n = 738)	At Home	83% (611)
	At Work	84% (618)
Started Using Internet (n = 718)	Mode	1995
Technology Use 5 or More Days Each Week	E-mail	86% (617)
	Listserv	27% (188)
	WWW	64% (456)

* valid percentages and frequencies

Barriers to Internet Use

Respondents were asked to identify how significant 11 potential barriers were to their Internet use. The distribution of respondents is presented in Table 3. Over one-third (39%) stated that lack of time to change current practice was *very significant* or *significant*. Whereas, almost two-thirds (65.7%) reported lack of technology access to not be a significant barrier to their Internet use. Respondents used an identical four-point Likert scale to report their reactions to 13 statements about potential problems with respect to Internet use. The distribution of respondents is presented in Table 4. Two problems approximately 8 out of 10 respondents either *strongly agreed* or *agreed* with were encountering links that did not work and took too long to download.

Beliefs Regarding Internet Use

Respondents used a four-point Likert-type scale (strongly agree to strongly disagree) to report their beliefs regarding 26 statements about using the Internet. The distribution of respondent beliefs is presented in Table 5. The majority of respondents *strongly agreed* or *agreed* that the Internet provided credible information (85.1%) and was easy to access (91.4%). Almost three out of four *disagreed* or *strongly disagreed* that the Internet was intimidating (73.1%).

TABLE 3. Health Educators' Perceived Barriers to Internet Use (n = 738)

	Very Significant	Significant	Somewhat Significant	Not Significant	Non-Response
How significant are the following barriers to your Internet use?					
Lack of appropriate hardware at home	14.6% (108)	14.6% (108)	18.8% (139)	48% (354)	3.9% (29)
Lack of appropriate hardware at work	10.8% (80)	10.4% (77)	14.2% (105)	59.5% (439)	5% (37)
Lack of appropriate software at home	12.9% (95)	13% (96)	18.7% (138)	50.4% (372)	5% (37)
Lack of appropriate software at work	8.9% (66)	9.9% (73)	16.4% (121)	58.7% (433)	6.1% (45)
Lack of access to technology	7% (52)	8% (59)	14.9% (110)	65.7% (485)	4.3% (34)
Lack of adequate funds	14.1% (104)	14.4% (106)	24.3% (179)	42.7% (315)	4.6% (34)
Lack of knowledge about the Internet	7.7% (57)	13.1% (97)	26.7% (197)	48.9% (361)	3.5% (26)
Lack of Internet training	5.6% (41)	14.8% (109)	32.4% (239)	43.5% (321)	3.8% (28)
Lack of awareness of the Internet's potential	7.6% (56)	16.5% (122)	26% (192)	45.7% (337)	4.2% (31)
Lack of time to change current practices	16.5% (122)	22.5% (166)	27.6% (204)	28.9% (213)	4.5% (33)
Lack of expectations for use of the Internet in my job	4.7% (35)	12.1% (89)	22.6% (167)	54.9% (405)	5.7% (42)

TABLE 4. Health Educators' Perceived Problems with Internet Use (n = 738)

	Strongly Agree	Agree	Disagree	Strongly Disagree	Non-Response
While using the Internet potential problems occur when:					
I am unable to efficiently organize the information I gather	6.6% (49)	34.7% (256)	45.8% (338)	6.4% (47)	6.5% (48)
I am unable to find a page that I know is out there	6.5% (48)	50.4% (372)	33.7% (249)	3.7% (27)	5.7% (42)
I am unable to return to a page I once visited	6.4% (47)	32.9% (243)	46.9% (346)	8.1% (60)	5.7% (42)
I am unable to determine where I am (i.e, "lost in cyberspace")	3.9% (29)	23.2% (171)	55.4% (409)	11.7% (86)	5.8% (43)
I encounter links that do not work	13.6% (100)	66.7% (492)	12.9% (95)	1.1% (8)	5.8% (43)
I encounter links that take me to unexpected places	11.5% (85)	54.3% (401)	26.4% (195)	1.1% (8)	6.6% (49)
I have problems with my browser (e.g., freezing up, getting disconnected)	11.5% (85)	42.7% (315)	35% (258)	5% (37)	5.8% (43)
I encounter sites that require me to register for them	23% (170)	60.7% (448)	9.3% (69)	1.2% (9)	5.7% (42)
I encounter sites that take too long to load	21.4% (158)	59.9% (442)	11.5% (85)	.8% (6)	6.4% (47)
I encounter sites that contain useless graphics	18.4% (136)	46.5% (343)	27.6% (204)	1.5% (11)	6% (44)
I encounter sites that want me to pay to access information	22% (162)	49.2% (363)	20.5% (151)	2.3% (17)	6.1% (45)
Advertising banners take too long to load	24.1% (178)	47.2% (348)	19.8% (146)	1.4% (10)	7.6% (56)
I encounter unsolicited and inappropriate sites (i.e., pornography)	17.9% (132)	33.9% (250)	34.6% (255)	6.8% (50)	6.9% (51)

Training

The survey asked several questions regarding formal and informal training survey participants had received using the Internet (i.e., e-mail, chatrooms, search engines, virtual libraries) as well as whether they had taken or were willing to take a Web-based or Web-enhanced class. The majority of the respondents had not taken a Web-enhanced class or training (76%) or a Web-based class or training (91%). However, 80% were willing to take "an entirely Web-based education class."

TABLE 5. Health Educators' Beliefs Regarding Internet Use (n = 738)

	Strongly Agree	Agree	Disagree	Strongly Disagree	Non-Response
Using the Internet . . .					
Provides credible health information	21.1% (156)	64% (472)	8.4% (62)	.8% (6)	5.7% (42)
Is easily accessible	39.8% (294)	51.6% (381)	3.1% (23)	.1% (1)	5.3% (36)
Allows for dissemination of information to others	35.2% (260)	53.3% (393)	6.1% (45)	.5% (4)	4.9% (36)
Increases the speed of finding information	45.7% (337)	41.9% (309)	7% (52)	.8% (6)	4.6% (34)
Removes distance as a potential barrier	45.9% (339)	45% (332)	3.8% (28)	.5% (4)	4.7% (35)
Is secure	3.1% (23)	36.9% (272)	45.4% (335)	8% (59)	6.6% (49)
Increases the risk of inaccurate information	19.2% (142)	57.3% (423)	16.5% (122)	1.6% (12)	5.3% (39)
Is difficult to navigate	3.99% (29)	20.69% (152)	60.29% (444)	9.29% (68)	6.19% (45)
Is frustrating	3.7% (27)	35.1% (259)	47.6% (351)	8.8% (65)	4.9% (36)
Is convenient	39.4% (291)	50.5% (373)	4.7% (35)	.3% (2)	5% (37)
Increases professional networks	34.3% (253)	52.8% (390)	6% (44)	1.2% (9)	5.7% (42)
Provides access to reputable information	19.1% (141)	67.5% (498)	7% (52)	.4% (3)	6% (44)
Is an alternative educational mode	22.6% (167)	64.5% (476)	6.5% (48)	.7% (5)	5.7% (42)
Increases job effectiveness	29.1% (215)	58.9% (435)	4.9% (36)	.5% (4)	6.5% (48)
Provides instant access to information	38.3% (283)	53.5% (395)	3.3% (24)	.3 (2)	4.6% (34)
Decreases interpersonal communication	13.7% (101)	47.6% (351)	30.8% (227)	3.1% (23)	4.9% (36)
Risks violation of privacy	13.3% (98)	63.8% (471)	16.1% (119)	.8% (6)	6% (44)
Is intimidating	2.2% (16)	19.9% (147)	56.4% (416)	16.7% (123)	4.9% (36)
Reduces paper use	29.5% (218)	43.5% (321)	18.3% (135)	4.3% (32)	4.3% (32)
Is impersonal	8.8% (65)	45% (332)	37.5% (277)	3.7% (27)	5% (37)
Provides too much information	10.3% (76)	28.7% (212)	46.5% (343)	8.9% (66)	5.6% (41)
Is costly (i.e., hardware/ software/phone)	7.9% (58)	40% (295)	41.5% (306)	5.4% (40)	5.3% (39)
Is time consuming	17.3% (128)	46.5% (343)	27.9% (206)	3% (22)	5.3% (39)
Is inexpensive	11% (81)	44.9% (331)	33.5% (247)	5.6% (41)	5.1% (38)
Finds old, outdated links	4.1% (30)	45.9% (339)	34.7% (256)	2.3% (17)	13% (96)
Is slow	4.3% (32)	45.8% (338)	38.6% (285)	3.3% (24)	8% (59)

Confidence in Using the Internet

When asked to indicate overall confidence in their use of the Internet, 71% indicated they were either "confident" or "very confident," and only 4% indicated they were "not confident at all." Nine out of ten reported being "comfortable" (14%) or "very comfortable" (80%) with using e-mail, and over three-fourths were "comfortable" or "very comfortable" with using search engines (78%) and the Internet (85%). Less than half reported being "comfortable" or "very comfortable" with virtual libraries (48%), newsgroups (36%), discussion groups (28%), and chatrooms (27%). Overall, one-fifth (22%) were "very satisfied" with their current Internet skills, 59% were "somewhat satisfied," and only 3% of respondents were "very unsatisfied."

Channels of Information

When asked how they found out about new Internet pages/sites, over three-fourths of the respondents found them through friends (81%), by following links (82%), and using an Internet search engine (74%). Magazines, newspapers, and professional journals were listed by over 50% of the respondents as a means for finding new Websites. Fewer respondents heard about new Websites through television (38%), radio (23%) or billboards (13%).

Factor Analysis

The 11 items in the "Barriers to Internet Use" section were subjected to an exploratory factor analysis (Table 6). Inspection of the initial findings suggested a two-factor structure, and two factors were retained for rotation. Six items loaded on the first factor and four items loaded on the second factor. Next, the 26 items in the "Beliefs Regarding Internet Use" section were analyzed. Inspection of the initial findings suggested a three-factor structure, and three factors were retained for rotation. Ten items loaded on the first factor, four items the second factor, and three items loaded on the third factor. Finally, the 13 items in the "Potential Problems" section were analyzed using exploratory factor analysis. Inspection suggested a two-factor structure, and two factors were retained for rotation. Seven items loaded on the first factor, and four items on the second factor.

TABLE 6. Factor Analysis of Barriers, Potential Problems and Beliefs Toward Internet Use

Perceived Barriers to Internet Use	
Factor 1: Adequate Access (41.8%)	Lack of appropriate hardware at home (.55)
	Lack of appropriate hardware at work (.81)
	Lack of appropriate software at home (.54)
	Lack of appropriate software at work (.84)
	Lack of access to technology (.72)
	Lack of adequate funds (.67)
Factor 2: Training and Time (16.6%)	Lack of knowledge about the Internet (.86)
	Lack of Internet training (.93)
	Lack of awareness of the Internet's potential (.68)
	Lack of time to change current practices (.50)
Perceived Problems with Internet Use	
Factor 1: Website Problems (32.6%)	I encounter links that do not work (.44)
	I encounter sites that require me to register for them (.59)
	I encounter sites that take too long to load (.72)
	I encounter sites that contain useless graphics (.66)
	I encounter sites that want me to pay to access information (.59)
	Advertising banners take too long to load (.67)
	I encounter unsolicited and inappropriate sites (i.e., pornography) (.43)
Factor 2: Inability to Effectively Use (13.9%)	I am unable to efficiently organize the information I gather (.62)
	I am unable to find a page that I know is out there (.70)
	I am unable to return to a page I once visited (.74)
	I am unable to determine where I am (i.e., "lost in cyberspace") (.71)
Beliefs Toward Internet Use	
Factor 1: Relative Advantage (20.8%)	Provides credible health information (.53)
	Is easily accessible (.57)
	Allows for dissemination of information to others (.57)
	Increases the speed of finding information (.54)
	Removes distance as a potential barrier (.50)
	Is convenient (.62)
	Increases professional networks (.54)
	Provides access to reputable information (.64)
	Is an alternative educational mode (.52)
	Increases job effectiveness (.60)
	Provides instant access to information (.73)
Factor 2: Relative Disadvantage (9.6%)	Is secure ($-.46$)
	Increases the risk of inaccurate information (.47)
	Decreases interpersonal communication (.40)
	Risks violation of privacy (.59)
Factor 3: Complexity (6.7%)	Is difficult to navigate (.49)
	Is frustrating (.68)
	Is intimidating (.59)

Study Limitations

There are potential limitations to the study that should be considered when reviewing results and drawing conclusions. The findings are based on self-report data and may be subject to recall bias. Results from this study are only generalizable to those health educators who were Certified Health Education Specialists (CHES) and/or were listed in the Health Education Directory (HEDIR) in the fall of 1999. Non-respondents, who were in the electronic mail survey group, may have been less Internet savvy or felt uncomfortable with the technology, and therefore, did not respond, biasing the overall sample.

IMPLICATIONS FOR THE PROFESSION

Today, many Internet resources are health-related, and researching health information is one of the most popular reasons for using the Internet (Eng et al., 1998). The Internet's importance was also recognized by a panel of health education experts when accessing online health information resources was established as one of its stated sub-competencies under the entry-level responsibility for a health educator acting as a resource person in health education (National Commission for Health Education Credentialing, Inc., 1996). Results from this survey are consistent with previous findings (Hanks et al., 2000), suggesting that the majority of health educators have embraced basic Internet practices (5+ days e-mail use, 86%; 5+ days World Wide Web use, 64%) and have access to the Internet (84%). The critical issue becomes whether they have the ability to effectively use the Internet to improve health education practice and research.

The survey results suggest that training to better understand how to most effectively use the Internet as a "tool" of the profession is needed. Hands-on workshops and one-on-one training may be difficult to provide on a large-scale basis to health educators already working in the field; however, over three-fourths of the respondents indicated they would be willing to take a Web-based course. This may be an opportunity for colleges and universities and/or professional organizations to provide online continuing education for practitioners to better understand the Internet and how to maximize its use.

The factor analysis can assist in understanding this group of health educators regarding motivators and barriers to Internet use. Adequate access, Website problems, and relative advantage are key factors that influence Internet use. Whereas, as complexity, relative disadvantage or inability to effectively use are not as significant factors. These factors need to be acknowledged during trainings and in professional preparation programs. If adequate access is a key issue from a software and hardware perspective, training health educators in technology applications that they cannot use in their jobs is frustrating and may decrease appropriate Internet use. Training should focus on how to overcome potential problems and focus on the relative advantages of the Internet (i.e., credible health information, easy access).

As health educators we use the basic principle of *starting where the people are* (Nyswander, 1956), we should do the same for ourselves. Develop trainings that are tailored to the needs of health educators recognizing the limitations that their workplace may impose upon their ability to incorporate all aspects of Internet technology.

Future research focusing on the adoption of the Internet is critical for the health education profession. Sultan and Chan (2000) present a model to distinguish between adopters and nonadopters based on several categories including the individual's perception of technology. A similar model could be used with health educators.

This study attempts to fill a void in the health education literature regarding Internet use, motivators and barriers among a select group of health educators. This first of its kind survey among health educators can help guide continuing education, university health education curriculums, and research agendas.

REFERENCES

Computer Industry Almanac (1999). U.S. tops 100 million Internet users according to Computer Industry Almanac [Online]. Available: http://www.c-i-a.com/, November 4, 1999 [2001, January 25].

Dillman, D.A. (2000). *Mail and Internet Surveys: The Tailored Design Method.* New York: John Wiley & Sons, Inc.

Eng, T.R., Maxfield, A., Patrick, K., Deering, M.J., Ratzan, S.C., & Gustafson, D.H. (1998). Access to health information and support: A public highway or private road? *Journal of the American Medical Association, 280,* 1371-1375.

Fulop, M.P., Loop-Bartick, K., & Rossett, A. (1997). Using the World Wide Web to conduct a needs assessment. *Performance Improvement, 36*(6), 22-27.

Hanks, W. A., Barnes, M.D., Merrill, R.M., & Neiger, B. (2000). Computer task and application use by professional health educators: Implications for professional preparation. *Journal of Health Education, 31*(6), 314-319.

Hatcher, L. (1994). *A Step-by-Step Approach to Using SAS® System for Factor Analysis and Structural Equation Modeling.* Cary, NC: SAS Institute, Inc.

Hollander, S.M., & Martin, E.R. (1999). Public health professionals in the Midwest: A profile of connectivity and information technology skills. *Bull Medical Library Association, 87,* 329-336.

Jackson, E.N., & Chun-Ju Chang, R. (2001). Click, click: Building Florida roads into the superhighway. *Florida Journal of Health, Physical Education, Recreation, Dance and Driver Education, 39,* 44-47.

Kittleson, M.J. (1999). A simple guide to putting evaluation assessments onto the web. *International Electronic Journal of Health Education, 2,* 94-100.

Kotecki, J.E., & Siegel, D. (1997). Finding health information via the WWW: An essential resource for the community health practitioner. *Journal of Health Education, 28,* 117-120.

Kraemer, H.C., & Thiemann, S. (1987). *How Many Subjects? Statistical Power Analysis in Research.* Newbury Park, CA: Sage Publications.

McCormack Brown, K.R. (2001). Using the Internet to access oral health information. *Journal of Dental Hygiene, 75,* 39-44.

McCormack Brown, K.R. (1998). Designing web-based experiences for health educators: A teaching idea for profession preparation. *Journal of Health Education, 29,* 373-375.

McDermott, R.J., & Sarvela, P.D. (1999). *Health Education and Measurement: A Practitioner's Perspective* (2nd ed.). Dubuque, IA: WC Brown.

McKenzie, J.F., Wood, M.L., Kotecki, J.E., Clark, J.K., & Brey, R.A. (1999). Establishing content validity: Using qualitative and quantitative steps. *American Journal of Health Behavior, 23,* 311-318.

National Commission for Health Education Credntialing, Inc. (1996). *A Competency-Based Framework for Professional Development of Certified Health Education Specialists.* Allentown, PA: NCHEC.

Nicholson, T., Duncan, D., & White, J.B. (1999). A survey of adult recreational use via the WWW: The DRUGNET study. *Journal of Psychoactive Drugs, 31,* 415-422.

Nicholson, T., White, J., & Duncan, D. (1998). Drugnet: A pilot study of adult recreational drug use via the WWW. *Substance Abuse, 19,* 109-121.

Nyswander, D. (1956). Education for health: Some principles and their application. *Health Education Monographs, 14,* 65-70.

Pealer, L.N., & Weiler, R.M (2000). Web-based health survey research: A prime. *American Journal of Health Behavior, 24*(1), 69-72.

Perrin, K.M., & Mayhew, D. (2000). The reality of designing and implementing an Internet-based course. *Journal of Distance Learning Administration, 3*(4), 12-15.

Powell, J., & Clarke, A. (2002). The WWW of the world wide web: Who, what, and why? *Journal of Medical Internet Research, 4*(1), e4.

Randolfi, E.A. (1998). Teaching online consumer health skills. *International Electronic Journal of Health Education, 1*(4), 201-206.

Reneau, J., Nicholson, T., White, J.B., & Duncan, D. (2000). The general well-being of recreational drug-users: A survey on the WWW. *International Journal of Drug Policy, 11,* 315-323.

Sultan., F., & Chan, L. (2000). The adoption of new technology: The case of object-oriented computing in software companies. *IEEE Transactions on Engineering Management, 47,* 106-126.

Turner, J.L., & Turner, D.B. (1998). Using the Internet to perform survey research. *Syllabus,* 58-61.

Beyond the Individual: Environmental Approaches and Prevention, edited by Abraham Wandersman, PhD, and Robert E. Hess, PhD* (Vol. 4, No. 1/2, 1985). *"This excellent book has immediate appeal for those involved with environmental psychology . . . likely to be of great interest to those working in the areas of community psychology, planning, and design." (Australian Journal of Psychology)*

Prevention: The Michigan Experience, edited by Betty Tableman, MPA, and Robert E. Hess, PhD* (Vol. 3, No. 4, 1985). *An in-depth look at one state's outstanding prevention programs.*

Studies in Empowerment: Steps Toward Understanding and Action, edited by Julian Rappaport, Carolyn Swift, and Robert E. Hess, PhD* (Vol. 3, No. 2/3, 1984). *"Provides diverse applications of the empowerment model to the promotion of mental health and the prevention of mental illness." (Prevention Forum Newsline)*

Aging and Prevention: New Approaches for Preventing Health and Mental Health Problems in Older Adults, edited by Sharon P. Simson, Laura Wilson, Jared Hermalin, PhD, and Robert E. Hess, PhD* (Vol. 3, No. 1, 1983). *"Highly recommended for professionals and laymen interested in modern viewpoints and techniques for avoiding many physical and mental health problems of the elderly. Written by highly qualified contributors with extensive experience in their respective fields." (Clinical Gerontologist)*

Strategies for Needs Assessment in Prevention, edited by Alex Zautra, Kenneth Bachrach, and Robert E. Hess, PhD* (Vol. 2, No. 4, 1983). *"An excellent survey on applied techniques for doing needs assessments. . . . It should be on the shelf of anyone involved in prevention." (Journal of Pediatric Psychology)*

Innovations in Prevention, edited by Robert E. Hess, PhD, and Jared Hermalin, PhD* (Vol. 2, No. 3, 1983). *An exciting book that provides invaluable insights on effective prevention programs.*

Rx Television: Enhancing the Preventive Impact of TV, edited by Joyce Sprafkin, Carolyn Swift, PhD, and Robert E. Hess, PhD* (Vol. 2, No. 1/2, 1983). *"The successful interventions reported in this volume make interesting reading on two grounds. First, they show quite clearly how powerful television can be in molding children. Second, they illustrate how this power can be used for good ends." (Contemporary Psychology)*

Early Intervention Programs for Infants, edited by Howard A. Moss, MD, Robert E. Hess, PhD, and Carolyn Swift, PhD* (Vol. 1, No. 4, 1982). *"A useful resource book for those child psychiatrists, paediatricians, and psychologists interested in early intervention and prevention." (The Royal College of Psychiatrists)*

Helping People to Help Themselves: Self-Help and Prevention, edited by Leonard D. Borman, PhD, Leslie E. Borck, PhD, Robert E. Hess, PhD, and Frank L. Pasquale* (Vol. 1, No. 3, 1982). *"A timely volume . . . a mine of information for interested clinicians, and should stimulate those wishing to do systematic research in the self-help area." (The Journal of Nervous and Mental Disease)*

Evaluation and Prevention in Human Services, edited by Jared Hermalin, PhD, and Jonathan A. Morell, PhD* (Vol. 1, No. 1/2, 1982). *Features methods and problems related to the evaluation of prevention programs.*

Index

Numbers followed by "f" indicate figures; "t" following a page number indicates tabular material.